The Miracle at
Speedy Motors

The Miracle at
Speedy Motors

ALEXANDER McCALL SMITH

Little, Brown

LITTLE, BROWN

First published in Great Britain in 2008 by Little, Brown
Reprinted 2008 (four times)

Copyright © Alexander McCall Smith 2008

The moral right of the author has been asserted.

*All characters and events in this publication, other than those
clearly in the public domain, are fictitious and any resemblance
to real persons, living or dead, is purely coincidental.*

All rights reserved.
No part of this publication may be reproduced, stored in a
retrieval system, or transmitted, in any form or by any means, without
the prior permission in writing of the publisher, nor be otherwise circulated
in any form of binding or cover other than that in which it is published
and without a similar condition including this condition
being imposed on the subsequent purchaser.

A CIP catalogue record for this book
is available from the British Library.

Hardback ISBN 978-0-316-03007-6
C-format ISBN 978-0-316-03008-3

Typeset in Galliard by M Rules
Printed and bound in Great Britain by
Clays Ltd, St Ives plc

Little, Brown
An imprint of
Little, Brown Book Group
100 Victoria Embankment
London EC4Y 0DY

An Hachette Livre UK Company
www.hachettelivre.co.uk

www.littlebrown.co.uk

For my wife Elizabeth,
a kind doctor, a worker of miracles

Chapter One

We Are All Care
of One Another

The correct address of Precious Ramotswe, Botswana's foremost solver of problems – in the sense that this was where she could be found between eight in the morning and five in the afternoon, except when she was not there – was The No. 1 Ladies' Detective Agency, c/o Tlokweng Road Speedy Motors, Gaborone, Botswana. The 'care of' was a matter of some disagreement between Mma Ramotswe and Grace Makutsi, her assistant and 'right-hand lady', as she put it. Mma Makutsi, with all the dignity of one who had received ninety-seven per cent in the final examinations of the Botswana Secretarial College, took the view that to say that the agency

1

was *care of* Speedy Motors was to diminish its importance, even if it was true that the agency occupied a small office at the side of the garage. Those who really counted in this life, she maintained, were usually not *care of* anybody.

'We are the ones they come looking for,' she argued, with perhaps less than perfect logic. 'When people come to this place, Mma, they look for us, not for the garage. The garage customers all know where the garage is. So our name should be first in the address, not the other way round, Mma. If anything, *Speedy Motors* should be care of us.'

She looked at Mma Ramotswe as she said this, and then quickly added: 'That is not to say that Mr J. L. B. Matekoni and his garage are not important, Mma. That is not to say such a thing. It is just a question of . . .'

Mma Ramotswe waited for her assistant to complete the sentence, but nothing further came. That was the trouble with Mma Makutsi, she thought; she left things hanging in the air, often the most important things. What was it a question of? It must be a question of status, she decided; Mma Makutsi could be very prickly about that. There had been that business about her being described as 'senior secretary' when she had only been in the job for a couple of months and when there was nobody junior to her in the firm; in fact, when there was nobody else at all in the firm. Then, once she had been promoted to assistant detective, it had not been long before she had asked when she could expect to be an 'associate detective'. That promotion had come, as had her earlier advancement, at a time when Mma Ramotswe had been feeling guilty about something or other and had felt the need to smooth ruffled feathers. But now that she was an associate detective it was difficult to see what the next step could be. She had a suspicion that Mma Makutsi hankered after the title of 'chief detective' – a suspicion which was founded on Mma Ramotswe's having found in the waste-paper basket a crumpled piece of paper on which Mma Makutsi had been trying out new signatures. Not only were there several attempts at *Mma Grace Radiphuti*, Radiphuti being the surname of her fiancé, Phuti, but there was also a scrawled signature, *Grace Makutsi*, under which she had written *Chief Detective*.

Mma Ramotswe had re-crumpled the paper and tossed it back into the basket. She felt bad about having read it in the first place; one should not look uninvited at the papers of another, even if they had been discarded. And it was entirely understandable, normal even, that an engaged woman should practise the signature she will use after her marriage. Indeed, Mma Ramotswe suspected that most women secretly experimented with a new signature shortly after meeting a man they looked upon with favour – even if that man had not expressed any interest in them. A handsome and eligible man might expect to have his name tried out in this way by many women who fancied themselves on his arm, and there was no harm in this, she thought, unless one believed that women should not prepare quite so willingly for their hearts to be broken. Women, thought Mma Ramotswe, are sometimes like plump chickens in the yard, while outside, circling the fence, were the hyenas, the men. It was not a happy way of envisaging the relation between the sexes, but time and time again she had seen this particular drama played out in exactly that way. And hyenas, one had to admit, were surely destined to break the hearts of chickens; they could do nothing else.

Mma Ramotswe saw nothing undignified in being in the care of anybody. In fact, she thought it was rather reassuring to be in another's care and, more than that, it was a very convenient way of describing how to find somebody, a way which we used in our everyday lives when talking about those we knew. There were people who were always to be found in the company of one particular friend, and to say, 'Oh, you'll always find him walking around with that other man, you know, the one who lives next to the store,' was surely the same as saying that one was care of the other. Yes, we were all care of one another in the final analysis, at least in Botswana, where people looked for and valued those invisible links that connected people, that made for belonging. We were all cousins, even if remote ones, of somebody; we were all friends of friends, joined together by bonds that you might never see, but that were there, sometimes every bit as strong as hoops of steel.

But, Mma Ramotswe thought that morning as she drank her first cup of red bush tea during her walk about her garden, perhaps this did not apply to everybody; perhaps there were some who were lonely in the middle of all this profusion of friends and relatives, who had lost their people. And that very morning, she would be seeing a woman who had written to her with exactly that problem, a woman who wanted to trace her relatives. Tracing people was bread and butter to some-body in Mma Ramotswe's profession; at least once a month someone would come into the office and ask her to find some-body – an errant husband, a lover, a child who had drifted away from the family and stopped writing home. Sometimes it was lawyers who contacted her and asked her to find those who stood to inherit cattle, or land, and did not know of the good fortune that awaited them. That was the sort of case that Mma Ramotswe most enjoyed, and when she succeeded in finding such people, as she usually did, she relished the moment when she disclosed to them what was in store. Earlier that week she had found a young man who did not know that his uncle in the north had died and left him three trucks and a taxi. She had forgiven him the speed with which his expression of sorrow at the news of the uncle's demise was replaced by one of incredulity and then joy when he heard of the vehicles await-ing him under a shade-netting awning somewhere up in Maun. Young men were human, after all, and this young man, she learned, had been saving to build a small house for himself and his bride-to-be. He needed to save no more.

'Three trucks, did you say, Mma? What make?'

Mma Ramotswe had no idea. Trucks were Mr J. L. B. Matekoni's concern, not hers. She was not even sure she could identify the manufacturer of her tiny white van; there had been a name painted on the back at one stage but over the years it had been obliterated by the wind and clouds of dust and the scratching of thorn bushes. Now there was nothing, just ridges in the metal where there had been letters. Not that it mattered,

5

of course: the tiny white van was too old to remember its maker, too ancient to be taken back.

Missing names, missing persons – how remarkable it was, she thought, that we managed to anchor ourselves at all in this world, and that we did so by giving ourselves names and linking those names with places and other people. But there were people, she imagined, whose names said nothing about them and who had only the haziest idea of who they were, people who might never even have known their parents. Mma Ramotswe could not remember her mother, who died when she was a baby, but at least she had known her father, the late Obed Ramotswe, whose memory seemed undimmed by the passage of the years. She thought of him every day, every day, and believed that in due course – but not too soon, she hoped – she would see him again in that place that was Botswana but not Botswana, that place of gentle rain and contented cattle. And perhaps on that day those people who had nobody here would find that there were indeed people for them. Perhaps.

Mma Ramotswe arrived in the office slightly before Mma Makutsi that morning. In the next-door premises of Tlokweng Road Speedy Motors, her husband, Mr J. L. B. Matekoni, was already hard at work with his two apprentices. Or rather, Mr J. L. B. Matekoni was hard at work; the apprentices gave the appearance of busying themselves with the servicing of a car but were more concerned with chatting about their activities of the previous evening. Charlie, the older of the two, and the ringleader, as Mr J. L. B. Matekoni thought of him, had recently moved into a room in a shared house in Old Naledi and was regaling his younger colleague with tales of how suitable this room was for the entertaining of girlfriends.

'It's a great place to take them,' he said. 'It's tops. A1. They come in and see how nice it is and they say, "Wow! Is this where you live, Charlie?"' This last was uttered in a voice intended to sound like a girl's, a high-pitched, silly voice going up at the end and culminating in a squeak.

The younger apprentice laughed, but Mr J. L. B. Matekoni, glancing over from his task of cleaning an air filter, grimaced. 'Not all girls speak like that, you know,' he muttered. 'And it's a good thing that Mma Makutsi isn't around to hear you making fun of young women. I wouldn't like to be in your shoes if she heard you.'

'I'm not frightened of her, Boss,' Charlie sneered. 'She's just a woman. I'm not frightened of any woman.'

Mr J. L. B. Matekoni felt himself getting hot around the back of his neck; the encountering of such silliness always had that effect on him. I know I should not pay any attention to this nonsense, he told himself. Charlie is just a young man who knows nothing yet. I shouldn't allow myself . . . But it was not easy to listen to such a complete travesty of the truth and register no protest. Of course Charlie was afraid of Mma Makutsi – who wasn't? Even Mma Ramotswe had confessed to Mr J. L. B. Matekoni that there were times when she trod very carefully in the face of her assistant's disapproval.

'So you're not afraid of her?' he said. 'That's very interesting. And you say that she's just a woman. What does that
mean? That you're better than any woman?'

Charlie laughed. 'I didn't say that, Boss. It may be true, of
course, but I didn't say it. I know better than to say things like
that when there are all these women around these days.
Hundreds of them – all ready to chop your head off if you say
something they don't like. Chop! One time! Off! Even here in
Botswana.'

Mr J. L. B. Matekoni turned back to his work. There was no
point in engaging these young men in debate, and he had to
admit that there was an element of truth in Charlie's final
remark. Botswana was known for its tolerance of debate and
criticism; anybody could criticise anybody, even at weddings
and funerals, where there would often be long speeches in
which old, controversial business was dragged up. And women
loved that sort of thing and were often ready to launch into an
attack on some unfortunate man who had spoken out of turn.
Why, he wondered, could people not disagree in a courteous
way, rather than resorting to unkind criticism?

Inside the office, Mma Ramotswe heard nothing of this
exchange; all she heard was the mumble of the men talking
amongst themselves, about, she imagined, the sort of thing
that men liked to talk about – spare parts, hydraulic systems,
suspension. She looked at her watch, which she always kept ten
minutes fast for the reassurance of knowing that one always
had ten minutes in hand. The appointment with the client –

the one who had written the letter asking her to find her family – was in half an hour's time. If Mma Makutsi were to be late this morning, they would not have time to deal with the mail that she would pick up from the post box on her way in to the office. This would not matter a great deal, as they would have plenty of time to deal with it later. But Mma Ramotswe liked to have her letters written early so that she could concentrate on her clients without thinking of tasks that lay ahead.

When she arrived several minutes later, Mma Makutsi had four or five letters in her hand. She placed these, almost reverentially, on her employer's desk before she hung up her scarf and the over-the-shoulder handbag she had recently taken to carrying. Mma Ramotswe did not see the point of either of these accessories, but was too polite to mention it to her assistant. To begin with, the scarf was the wrong colour for Mma Makutsi – or was it the wrong design? Mma Makutsi had problematic skin – slightly blotchy – and the difficulty with this scarf was that it was spotted. Those with spots, thought Mma Ramotswe, should not *wear* spots; that, surely, was fairly obvious. But how did one convey this fashion truth to one who appeared to enjoy wearing spotted items, like this ill-chosen scarf? There were some who believed that one should be direct in such cases and say exactly what one was thinking. So one might say, 'A traditionally built person, like you, should not wear stripes that run across the way. Your stripes should go up and down.' That, at least, was direct, and unambiguous, but it could give offence, especially in these days when fewer people wished to be considered traditionally built.

9

Mma Ramotswe had never been able to understand that, and considered it one of the very worst features of modern society that people should be ashamed to be of traditional build, cultivating instead a look that was bony and positively uncomfortable. Everybody knows, she thought, that we have a skeleton underneath our skin; there's no reason to show it.

'We'll have to hurry, Mma,' said Mma Ramotswe, pointing at her watch. 'That lady is coming to see us in half an hour.'

'Forty minutes,' said Mma Makutsi. 'Half an hour plus ten minutes. Your watch, Mma—'

'No, I've already taken ten minutes off what my watch says. It's half an hour, Mma.'

Mma Makutsi shrugged. 'Well, it would be far better if they started to deliver mail in this country rather than simply throwing it into a post box. It takes me at least fifteen minutes to walk to the box and get the letters. Every day. That's over one hour every week spent in just picking up letters. That is a big waste of time.' She drew in her breath; she was warming to her theme. 'At the Botswana Secretarial College they said that we should work out how much time it takes to perform small tasks and then multiply it by five to see how much of the week it takes. Then multiply by four to see what it takes over the whole month.'

Mma Ramotswe nodded. 'Sometimes I think of the time it takes to make tea and then to drink it. It's four minutes to boil the water and then there is all the business of putting the tea in the pot—'

The issue of tea breaks took them onto dangerous ground,

and she was quickly interrupted by Mma Makutsi. 'That is quite different, Mma,' she said. 'I was talking about the mail. Why can't they deliver it? They do that in other countries, you know. If your house has a number, they bring the letter to you.'

Mma Ramotswe thought about this for a moment. Mma Makutsi certainly had a point; Tlokweng Road Speedy Motors had a plot number and provided the agency used this in its address, then the post office should be able to find them. But not everybody was in that position. Out in the villages, or even in some parts of Gaborone, things became higgledy-piggledy as people built their houses wherever they pleased. How would the post office deal with that? She raised this difficulty with Mma Makutsi who listened attentively, but then shook her head in disagreement.

'All they have to do is to get somebody who knows the district,' she said. 'That would be easy enough, especially in the villages. Everybody knows who's who in the villages. You don't need a plot number there.' She paused. 'And there's another thing – if you forgot somebody's name, all you would need to do would be to write a description of what they look like on the envelope. That would do.'

Mma Ramotswe glanced up at the ceiling. One of the plaster-boards was discoloured at the edges, where rain had made its way in during the previous rainy season, and would have to be replaced. Mma Makutsi was right about villages, even the bigger ones, like Mochudi, where Mma Ramotswe had been born. Those places were still intimate enough for a rough

11

description to suffice. If somebody had written a letter addressed to 'That man who wears the hat, the one who was a miner and knows a lot about cattle, Mochudi, Botswana', it would undoubtedly have been correctly delivered to her father.

'Yes,' said Mma Ramotswe. 'I think you're right. But I don't think that they will ever do it. You know how governments are – always wanting to save money . . .'

She stopped. Her eye had caught the envelope on the top of the small pile of letters brought in by Mma Makutsi. It was addressed: To the lady detective, Tlokweng Road, Gaborone. That was all, but somewhere in the post office an obliging clerk had scrawled her box number in red ink. It was an extraordinary coincidence, and Mma Makutsi burst out laughing when she saw the envelope.

'Well, there you are, Mma,' she said. 'They can find people if they want to.'

They looked at the envelope. The address was written in capital letters, as if by a child, or one who found writing difficult. Anybody can contact us, Mma Ramotswe thought, even those who have little education, or are frightened; people at the bottom of the heap. We will turn nobody away, nobody.

She reached for the letter opener and slid its blade under the flap of the envelope. Inside was a flimsy piece of paper torn, it seemed, from a cheap notebook. She unfolded it and held it up to the light.

Fat lady: you watch out! And you too, the one with the big glasses. You watch out too!

She let the paper drop to the floor. Sensing that something was wrong, Mma Makutsi stepped forward and picked up the letter and read it out loud.

'There's no signature,' she said simply. 'Where can I file it if there is no signature?'

Chapter Two

A Woman of No Family

You simply have to put some things out of your mind, Mma Ramotswe told herself as Mma Makutsi ushered the client into the office. Mma Makutsi's reaction to the anonymous letter had been exemplary. She had read out the contents in a voice that remained resolutely level and then, without any comment, had raised the issue of where the letter might be filed. That was more than mere coolness of head – that was bravery, especially since the letter-writer had included Mma Makutsi in his crude threat.

She assumed that it was a man, as such a letter would never have been written by a woman. It was not that women never threatened physical violence – they did, even if not as readily as men did. One of the giveaways, as far as Mma Ramotswe was concerned, was the way in which she herself had been described. One woman would not describe another as ... *traditionally built* in that insulting way. All women knew that traditional build was something that could happen to anyone, and would not abuse another for it. Nor would a woman single out another woman's glasses for dismissive attention; hair and skin were the things a spiteful woman would notice – not glasses. No, the writer of the letter was a man, and a man who was, she suspected, consumed by envy. Nobody but an envious person, she thought, would write an anonymous letter of that sort.

Mma Ramotswe was still feeling shocked when Mma Makutsi, who had tucked the letter into an open file at the front of the cabinet, noticed the car drawing up outside.

'That lady is early,' she observed. 'She is parking next to your van. She is trying to get a bit of shade for her car.'

Mma Ramotswe pulled herself together. She would put the letter out of her mind and give her full attention to her client. Letters like that were best ignored. Their writers wanted one to worry – that was the whole point of writing them. They never meant any of the threats they made; if they really wanted to harm somebody, then they went ahead and did it. Threateners threatened; doers did.

Now, standing up behind her desk, as she always did when a client entered the room, Mma Ramotswe reached out to shake hands with the woman who had written that other, quite different letter to her.

'My name is Manka Sebina,' said the woman. 'You have not met me before, Mma, but I have seen you. I have seen you over at that fabric store in the African mall. I have seen you going in there.'

Mma Ramotswe laughed good-naturedly. 'This is a small town still,' she said. 'You cannot go out without being seen! And it is always when you're doing something like shopping or treating yourself to a doughnut. That is when you're seen. You're never seen when you're doing something good, like going to church.'

The woman sat down. 'But I have seen you doing that too, Mma,' she said. 'I have seen you going into the Anglican cathedral opposite the hospital. And I saw you outside after the service once. Drinking tea with Bishop Mwamba.'

Mma Ramotswe stared at her visitor, bemused. 'Perhaps you should be a detective yourself, Mma,' she said. As she spoke, she glanced in Mma Makutsi's direction, wondering what her assistant made of this. Was it nosiness? Or was it something else? There were people who took an excessive interest in the affairs of others, of people whom they did not know – stalkers, they were called. Mma Ramotswe wondered whether she had by unfortunate chance acquired a stalker and whether this woman sitting before her could be the person who had written the anonymous letter . . . in which case the man who had written the letter was really a woman after all.

Mma Sebina smiled nervously. 'No, please do not misunderstand me, Mma. I was not looking out for you specially. It's just that here in Gaborone we can't help but notice people who stand out.' She met Mma Ramotswe's eyes directly, but only for a short time before her gaze fell away. That was the way it was in Botswana – one engaged sideways, one did not stare in a direct and challenging way. Mma Sebina was well brought up, obviously; she knew. 'And you see, Mma, you are the only lady detective in this town. That is why everybody knows who you are. They say, "She is the detective, that woman. There she is."'

Mma Ramotswe's suspicions quickly evaporated. What Mma Sebina said was undoubtedly true. There were many people in Gaborone who had a completely unrealistic idea of what a private detective did, and imagined that she was some sort of secret agent engaged in all sorts of dramatic goings-on. Whereas the reality was that her life was really rather mundane, involving routine inquiries that were often no more demanding or dramatic than looking in the telephone directory or checking up on debt judgements handed down by Gaborone magistrates' court. It was understandable, perhaps, that people with an unrealistic view of her job should notice her and pass comment, and it was harmless enough; after all, she noticed people and wondered what they were up to. Only the other day she had seen one of her neighbours coming out of a shop carrying four large red buckets and a coil of plastic hosing. She had wondered what he could possibly want four buckets for, and it had occurred to her that he might be thinking of brewing beer and starting an illegal drinking den, a shebeen. That would be appalling, if it happened, as shebeens attracted rowdy people in large numbers and it would be the end of all peace in Zebra Drive if a shebeen were to open up there.

But the business in hand was Mma Sebina, the woman sitting in front of her, not buckets and shebeens and the mysterious doings of neighbours. She looked at Mma Sebina and made a mental note of what she and Mma Makutsi called the *essential particulars*. They had not invented the term, having found it in the pages of her vade mecum, Clovis Andersen's *The Principles of Private Detection*. 'When you meet somebody for the first time,' wrote Clovis Andersen, 'make sure that you note the essential particulars. That means those aspects of their appearance which might be relevant to the case. You can ignore incidentals – the fact that a shoelace is frayed at the end or that there is a small stain on a jacket. That sort of thing is not an *essential particular* because a frayed shoelace or a stain on a piece of clothing tells us nothing about that person – they are things that can happen to anybody. But if a watch is worn on the right wrist rather than the left, if an item of clothing is particularly expensive, or if fingernails are bitten down to the quick, that can tell us something about who that person is, about what that person is like.'

Now, running a discreet eye up and down Mma Sebina – or up and down that part of her which was visible above the edge of her desk – Mma Ramotswe noted the neat, middle-cost clothing; the well-groomed but not ostentatiously braided hair; the carefully plucked eyebrows. This was a woman who took pride in her appearance, but was not driven by fashion.

And there was another thing that Mma Ramotswe noticed: Mma Sebina spoke with a certain reticence, which suggested that she was ready to stop if the person to whom she was speaking had something more important, more pertinent, to say. That was always a good sign, Mma Ramotswe thought. Too many people were determined to blurt out their views even if the person being addressed knew much more about the subject under discussion. Reticence was a good sign.

Mma Ramotswe straightened the pad before her on the desk and reached for a pencil. 'You wrote to me, Mma,' she said. 'You said that you hoped that I would be able to trace some family members for you. And the answer is yes, we can do that sort of thing. We are always doing it, aren't we, Mma Makutsi?'

Mma Sebina turned to look at Mma Makutsi, who smiled at her encouragingly. 'Yes,' said Mma Makutsi. 'We are experts at finding people, Mma. We have found many, many people – including some who did not want to be found.'

Mma Ramotswe nodded. 'Usually, though, we're looking for somebody who is quite happy to be found.' She paused. 'Tell me, Mma: who is this relative you are looking for?'

For a moment Mma Sebina looked puzzled, as if wondering why Mma Ramotswe should have missed something obvious. 'But I don't know, Mma. That's the whole point. I have come to see you because I do not know.'

'You do not know what, Mma?'

It was at this point that Mma Makutsi decided to intervene. 'She does not know the name of the relative. That can happen when a woman marries and changes her name. You may not meet the new husband and you may forget what his name is. It is easy to forget the name of a man.'

A short silence followed this remark. Mma Ramotswe did not object to her assistant's joining in a conversation with a client, but she rather wished that she would wait until asked for her opinion, as her interjections could sometimes distract the client and lead the conversation off in a strange direction. Mma Makutsi could also be tactless at times; on one occasion she had tut-tutted when a client had been telling Mma Ramotswe about something he had done. That had not helped, as the client had become sullen and taciturn, and Mma Ramotswe had been obliged to reassure him not only that everything he said in the office would remain confidential, but also that neither she nor Mma Makutsi would take it upon themselves to criticise his actions. 'It is not for us, Rra,' she had said, all the while looking at Mma Makutsi, 'to make you feel guilty. It is not for us.'

Mma Makutsi had nodded. 'God will do that,' she interjected. 'He is the one who will judge you.'

That had been an awkward consultation, and later Mma Ramotswe had felt obliged to discuss the issue with Mma Makutsi and remind her of the need for professional detachment. 'It is fully discussed by Mr Clovis Andersen in *The Principles of Private Detection*,' she had said. 'You should perhaps read that section, Mma. Mr Andersen says that you should not pass judgement on your client's behaviour. If you do that, the client might wonder if you are really on his side.'

Mma Makutsi had defended herself. 'But I was not passing judgement on him,' she said. 'I said that God would do that. You heard me, Mma. That is what I said.'

At least now there was no such exchange. Mma Makutsi's suggestion was reasonable enough – women did change their names when they married and that could cause confusion. But Mma Sebina was shaking her head.

'No,' she said. 'I don't think you understand me, Bomma. I have not forgotten the names of these people. I do not know who they are. I do not even know whether they exist, although I hope they do.'

Mma Ramotswe twirled the pencil round in her fingers. HB: medium-soft lead. It was the sort of pencil that tended to become blunt rather too quickly for her liking. Twirling a pencil, HB or otherwise, was helpful: it enabled one to do something while one was thinking.

'So you do not know who they are?' she mused. 'I suppose that can happen. If you have a very large family there must be cousins you don't know about. I think I might have such cousins somewhere.'

'Usually such relatives turn up when they need something,' ventured Mma Makutsi. 'Since I became engaged, Mma Sebina, I have found cousins who are very friendly. It is strange that they have not been friendly before, but now they must have realised that they wanted to be friendly all along.'

Mma Ramotswe decided that this would need a word of explanation. 'Mma Makutsi has recently become engaged to Mr Phuti Radiphuti,' she said. 'He is—'

'The owner of the Double Comfort Furniture Shop,' supplied Mma Sebina. 'I have seen him.'

Mma Ramotswe and Mma Makutsi exchanged glances. If it had been disconcerting for Mma Ramotswe to discover that Mma Sebina knew all about her, then it was now Mma Makutsi's turn to be surprised. But it was not discomfort that she felt, but a certain degree of pride that she was engaged to a man of position, and known to people, to strangers, as such. There were those who might laugh at Phuti's name, or indeed at the man himself; but he was a well-known businessman, and that counted for something.

'That is him,' she said. 'That is our store.'

Mma Ramotswe drew in her breath, momentarily shocked by Mma Makutsi's claim. She might be marrying into the Double Comfort Furniture Shop, but she was not yet the Double Comfort Furniture Shop itself. Indeed, technically the store still belonged to Phuti's father, even if the old man spent most of his time these days sleeping. You still own something when you are asleep, she felt like pointing out to Mma Makutsi, but did not. Mma Ramotswe was generous; if it meant so much to Mma Makutsi that she should be thought of as the owner of a store, then what harm was there in that? Her assistant had started life with nothing, or next to nothing, and if she now had something, then that was entirely due to hard work on her part. There had been the Botswana Secretarial College, where she had performed at a stellar level, and then there had been the dancing classes at which she had persisted with Phuti, a most unpromising dance partner, even when he trod on her toes and stammered so badly that she could hardly make out what he was trying to say. No, Mma Makutsi deserved every bit of status to which she laid claim; she deserved this far more than many of those more glamorous people did, those glamorous people who found that everything tumbled into their laps simply because they were good-looking or knew people who would help them. She knew of so many cases like that: the nephew of a chief finding a good job in Gaborone above those better qualified than he was; the son of a mining manager being given a job with a company that made parts for the mining industry; and so on. It had never been like that for Mma Makutsi.

Mma Sebina nodded. 'And it is a very fine store, Mma.' She turned back to face Mma Ramotswe. 'No, I wouldn't mind it at all if some cousins were to get in touch,' she continued. 'Even if they were greedy and just wanted money from me. I would still like to have some cousins. You see, Mma, I have no family.'

She spoke without self-pity, as one might observe that one had run out of tea, or small change, or something of that nature.

Mma Ramotswe put the pencil down on her desk. 'They are all late? That is terrible, Mma. That is very sad. These days—'

Mma Sebina raised a hand to stop her. 'No, it is not that. They are not late – or some of them are, but the others may or may not be. I don't know.' She paused. 'I should tell you my story, Mma Ramotswe. Then you will understand.'

Mma Ramotswe signalled to Mma Makutsi to put on the

kettle. The telling of a story, like virtually everything in this life, was always made all the easier by a cup of tea.

'What's the earliest you can remember?' began Mma Sebina. And then, without waiting for an answer, she continued: 'I can remember being four, Mma Ramotswe, but nothing before that. I can remember seeing a car in a ditch being pulled out by a tractor. And then the tractor ran over a chicken.

'Then I remember nothing else about being four, and suddenly I'm five and it is time to go to Sunday school. I was taken to Sunday school by my mother and she used to come back to fetch me hours later, or it seemed like hours. We were given little stamps which we stuck in our books. Pictures of Jesus walking on the water and things like that. I remember looking at that picture of the walking on the water for a long time – I loved it so much, and I still do, Mma. I still have that picture.'

Mma Ramotswe nodded. She understood. She, too, had pictures that she loved: her picture, printed on a plate, of Sir Seretse Khama, the first President of Botswana, that great man; she loved that picture because the expression on his face said so much to her. It was a gentle face, the face of a man who believed in his country and had stood up for what it represented, which was decency above all else; just that – decency. When she looked at that picture, it was as if he was still there: the late President, still watching over his country. And how proud he would be if he really could see it today, she thought; how proud.

'For most people it doesn't matter if they forget what happened before they were four,' Mma Sebina continued. 'That is because they know that it was not very much. But in my case it's different, Mma. That's when everything happened. But I cannot remember any of it.

'I can see that you're puzzled, Mma, and I can understand why. My mother, you see, the lady I called my mother a little bit earlier – she was not really my mother. I was the daughter of another woman altogether and that kind lady, my mother, and her kind husband, my father, who was not really my father, took me in and raised me as their own child.

'That, of course, is a very common thing, Mma. There are many people who are the child of one mother but raised by another. Their mother may become late – that is a very common reason for this sort of thing – or may be too poor to bring up children. There are many reasons why a sister or an aunt may bring up the child of another woman. Or a grandmother, of course. As you know, that is not at all unusual.'

She paused, and Mma Ramotswe, reaching for her pencil, sighed. 'It is almost the rule, these days, Mma. What with this illness and everything. Where would we be without the grandmothers?'

Mma Sebina agreed. 'You are right. The grandmothers are the pillars. They are the ones. But most of these children who are brought up by the grandmothers know who they are. They know that their grandmother is their grandmother and that their mother was such-and-such and their father was this man or that man. But I do not know even the brothers and sisters

25

of the kind people who brought me up. I know nothing, Mma. Nothing.' She looked down at the floor; the composure that she had shown earlier on was slipping. Now there was a note to her voice that suggested that not far beneath the surface there was a well of emotion and, beyond that, tears. 'I do not have a birth certificate, Mma. I do not even have that.'

Mma Ramotswe raised an eyebrow. 'So what do you have on your omang?' All Batswana had an omang, the identity card which established their citizenship. The Setswana word *omang* meant *who?* and that was the question which the omang answered.

'My omang says that I was born on the thirtieth of September,' said Mma Sebina. 'I used to be proud of that. I used to be proud of the fact that my birthday was the same day as Botswana Day, that I was born on the same day as our country. But now I know that this is just because they did not know when my real birthday was. So you see, Mma, I would like you to find me a birthday. Please find me a birthday, and find me some people.'

There was a silence. Outside, from the branches of the acacia tree under which Mma Ramotswe parked her tiny white van, there came the cooing of the ubiquitous Cape doves. Mma Ramotswe saw them through the window, in the corner of her eye, the two doves, who were lovers; Mma Dove, Rra Dove, as she and Mma Makutsi called them, symbols of faithfulness, and of belonging. *Find me a birthday. Find me some people.*

'Can you not ask those two good people?' she asked.

'Can you not ask the people who were mother and father to you?'

'They are late,' said Mma Sebina. 'They are both late.'

'I see.'

'And they never told me themselves. It was only after they became late that I heard. I heard it from the nurse who looked after my mother when she was very ill. She said: "Your mother was very sad. She told me that there was something she had wanted to talk to you about, but she had never managed to do so. She thought that you should know."'

Mma Ramotswe frowned. 'Why did she think that, Mma?'

Mma Sebina sighed. 'I have asked myself that time and time again. And I do not know the answer. Maybe it is because at the end, at the very end, people want the truth to be known. Maybe it is that.'

Mma Ramotswe uttered a tiny sound, a clicking of the tongue that almost became the drawn-out *ee* that signified yes in Setswana; almost.

'But I think,' went on Mma Sebina, 'that the more likely reason is that she wanted me to know so that she could help me to find my real family. And then she became late before she could talk to me about it.'

Yes, thought Mma Ramotswe. That is probably it. We keep secrets until we no longer have the breath to utter them, and then they go to the grave with us. And what, she wondered, would her secrets be; the very question, as it happened, that was going through Mma Makutsi's mind at the same time: what would Mma Ramotswe's secrets be? they *both* thought.

27

Chapter Three

Mr J. L. B. Matekoni
is Given a Cake

Nothing more was said about the anonymous letter that day, and by the time Mma Ramotswe left the office that evening she had almost forgotten it. It crossed her mind briefly, though, as she turned her car into Zebra Drive. Mma Sebina's earlier remark about her visit to the fabric shop – one of her favourite places, one of her few self-indulgences – had made her wonder how many other people knew details of her private life. Mma Sebina herself was not in the least bit threatening, and it did not matter what she knew, but what if the writer of that letter, that clearly unpleasant person, was aware of where she lived? She felt a sudden discomfort. What if that person, whoever he was, was watching her right now? She glanced into the mirror as she turned the corner. There was a car not far behind her, a nondescript white car of the sort that streamed out of office car parks in their hundreds come five o'clock in the afternoon; just as she started to turn, it signalled its intention of doing the same thing, and made to enter Zebra Drive.

Mma Ramotswe put her foot down on the accelerator. The tiny white van was not powerful; in fact, its engine, valiant though it might once have been, found great difficulty in coping even with normal demands. Now, with the encouragement of its driver, the van struggled to put on a bit of speed, and succeeded – to an extent. Mma Ramotswe again looked in her rear-view mirror and saw that the car behind her had also speeded up. That, she felt, settled the matter: she was being followed.

Her first thought, which was a resolution really, was not to panic. She had been a private detective for some years now and she had never considered herself to be in any real danger. Only once had she felt that she was in the presence of real evil, and that was when she had encountered Charlie Gotso BA. She had realised then that she was face to face with one who could deliberately dispose of somebody without a second thought. The realisation had appalled her, but she had not felt threatened herself. Now, though, she was being followed, and she felt fear. It was a taste in her mouth, a sound in her ears, a feeling on her skin.

She thought quickly. She was now not far from her driveway and her first inclination was to steer straight in and shut the gate firmly behind her. Her house was her sanctuary and there were people about – neighbours who were always watching what was going on and would answer any call for help. But then it occurred to her that if she did this, then she would be showing whoever it was who was following her that this was where she lived. That would not do, and indeed Clovis Andersen said something about this in *The Principles of Private Detection*; his words came back to her, as they often did in a crisis. *If you find you are being followed, never take the tail to your original destination; that is exactly what he wants! Go somewhere public. Stop. Get out of the car.*

It was good advice and she did not even slow down as she passed her house. The car behind her was keeping its distance, she noticed, and it kept that distance while she tried to decide what to do when she reached the end of Zebra Drive. If she turned left, she would end up driving past the hospital and the cathedral, and could eventually head back to the Tlokweng Road; if she opted to go right, then she would come out on the road that led to the flyover and the Francistown Road. There was always a great deal of traffic on that road and there was a chance that she could throw the other car off there, but she would have to stop sometime, and she felt more at home on this side of town. She could even stop outside Mma Makutsi's house, if need be, and invoke the help of her assistant and Phuti Radiphuti, if he was there. Not that Phuti would be much good, she thought; he was a kind man, and a gentle one, but she doubted whether he would be able to deal with the situation if it turned nasty.

She decided to go to the left. As she approached the end of
the road, she slowed down; the car behind her did not, and
Mma Ramotswe had to move swiftly off to avoid being
bumped into. She hardly dared look in her mirror as, hunched
over the steering wheel, the ancient engine of the tiny white
van straining every metal sinew, she careered down the road in
the direction of the hospital. At the roundabout, she threw the
vehicle with vigour into the circling traffic, narrowly missing a
truck, which sounded its horn angrily. 'I'm very sorry, Rra,' she
muttered under her breath. 'I am being chased. That is the
only reason why I'm driving like this.'

She had now passed the Anglican cathedral and was alongside the piece of ground used as a school playing field; hardly
a field, just a large square of level red earth, kicked into dust
here and there by the feet of the children. Mma Ramotswe
noticed that there were small boys running about; two teams
in identical khaki trousers and blue shirts, mostly barefoot,
were pursuing a dusty football. A match was in progress. She
saw the parents, lined up along the edge, shouting support for
their sons.

She saw her chance, and turned the tiny white van sharply
off the road, pointing it at a parking place between two
parental vehicles on the verge. She would be perfectly safe
here, amongst all these people, some of whom she was bound
to know. Clovis Andersen, she thought, would approve.

The car behind her stopped halfway off the road. Mma
Ramotswe watched in her mirror as it drew level with her. She
held her breath; she had not expected such effrontery, not

from somebody described in *The Principles of Private Detection* as a *tail*. Tails, surely, would be more discreet, fading off into the background when one stopped and looked at them.

The car had slightly tinted windows, which made it difficult to see the face of the person at the wheel. But now, directly behind the tiny white van, preventing it from returning to the road had Mma Ramotswe wished to do so, the car revealed its driver.

'Mma Ramotswe,' shouted a voice. 'I was trying to catch you! I've got something for you.'

She glanced in the mirror and then turned round in shock. Through the driver's window, now fully wound down, she could make out the familiar figure of Mma Potokwani, matron of the orphan farm, gesticulating frantically.

Mma Ramotswe took a deep breath. She knew that in a moment or two she would see the humour in the situation, but not just yet. A good minute had passed by the time she opened the door of the van and made her way towards Mma Potokwani's car.

'My goodness, Mma,' shouted Mma Potokwani. 'You were driving like one of those young men from the garage. What was the hurry?'

Mma Ramotswe did not answer; she had her own questions to ask, and they came tumbling out. 'And why are you driving that car, Mma Potokwani? How was I to know it was you? I thought that I was being followed by some . . . some . . .' She faltered. Some Tsotsi? Kidnapper? Writer of anonymous letters?

Mma Potokwani let out a hoot of laughter. 'Followed? Of

course I was following you. I saw you just before you turned into Zebra Drive. I saw your van. I wanted to give you something that I've made for Mr J. L. B. Matekoni. And this car – it belongs to one of the volunteers. They let me use it whenever I like.'

Mma Ramotswe forced a smile. 'It was silly of me,' she said. 'I just thought . . . You know, with my work, Mma, I sometimes get threats.'

Mma Potokwani frowned. 'People threaten you, Mma Ramotswe? Why would anybody want to threaten you?'

It was difficult to explain, particularly standing there in the late afternoon heat. And Mma Ramotswe thought that Mma Potokwani had little idea of what was involved in running a detective agency. She knew everything there was to know about managing an orphan farm, about getting things for the children, about cajoling supporters into donating, about making do with whatever she could purloin; but she knew nothing about the world of a detective agency.

'Sometimes I have to look into the affairs of people who don't want me to do so,' she explained. 'People can get angry.'

Mma Potokwani shrugged. 'We all get angry. I get angry with my husband from time to time, but I don't *follow* him.' She laughed. 'Perhaps wives should follow their husbands occasionally, though, just to see what they get up to. Perhaps it's a good idea, Mma Ramotswe.'

The matron now reached over the back of her seat to retrieve a large tin from the back of the car. 'This is for your husband, Mma. You can guess what it is.'

Mma Ramotswe could. And she knew too that the large, heavy fruit cake that the tin would contain would be more than a mere present: it would be a cake with a purpose. Mma Potokwani had always relied on Mr J. L. B. Matekoni for help with mechanical problems at the orphan farm – particularly with the old pump, but also with vehicles, cookers, water systems, and indeed anything that involved moving parts. He had always given this help without complaint, even if the tasks that he was called upon to perform took up a great deal of his spare time. But that was what he was like, and she was proud of him for it.

She knew that this present of a cake was a prelude to a major imposition on her husband. Really! One would have thought that Mma Potokwani would grasp that others could see through her obvious tricks, but she seemed utterly impervious to any hints along these lines.

'He will be very pleased,' she said. 'He loves your fruit cake. I wish I could make it as well as you do, Mma.'

Mma Potokwani clearly appreciated the compliment. 'You could learn, Mma. Maybe one day I shall teach you.' She passed the tin through the open window. 'Well, there you are, Mma. And perhaps, after he's eaten the cake, Mr J. L. B. Matekoni might like to bring the tin back to me. It's an old tin, but at least I could refill it for him if he brought it out.'

Mma Ramotswe smiled. That would be the way in which Mma Potokwani ensnared him; it was so obvious. 'Yes, of course,' she said. 'And he could take a look at things while he's out there . . .'

Mma Potokwani lost no time in seizing the opportunity. 'That's very kind of you, Mma. As a matter of fact, there are some things that could do with a bit of attention. There is a washing machine that we bought second-hand but paid good money for – two hundred pula, in fact. It seems to have given up now, but I'm sure it's just a little thing. And then there's the tractor, the small one. One of the men has done something to it and it will only go backwards now. I'm sure that Mr J. L. B. Matekoni would be able to sort that out in no time at all . . .'

'I'm sure he would,' said Mma Ramotswe. 'I shall tell him.'

Mma Potokwani gave a cheerful wave and began to drive off. There was a terrible grinding of gears as she did so; a noise like that which would be produced if a knife or a fork were to be put into a mincing machine. Mma Potokwani, though, seemed unconcerned. She waved again from the car and crashed the gears once more before moving off down the road in the direction of Tlokweng and the waiting orphans.

That evening, in the house on Zebra Drive, Mma Ramotswe and Mr J. L. B. Matekoni sat out on the verandah after dinner, reviewing the events of the day. The two foster children, Motholeli and Puso, were safely in bed. Motholeli, being older, was allowed to turn her own light out after she had finished reading, provided that it was off by half past nine; Puso's light had to be out an hour earlier than that, not that this was ever an issue with him. Like most boys, he spent his days in the relentless expenditure of energy, with the result that even by seven o'clock, when Mma Ramotswe placed the family meal on the table, he was tired to the point of exhaustion. Often Mma Ramotswe would go into his room a few minutes after the evening meal, drawing in her breath to deliver a homily on the need to tidy up the mess, only to discover the small boy lying, fully clad, on top of his blankets, already asleep.

She would gaze at him, at the perfection of his features – for he was an attractive child, with the honey-coloured skin of the Bushman side of his family, his mother and her people, but the taller build of his Motswana father. It was a good combination, a happy mixture. His Kalahari ancestors had bequeathed him eyes that shone with light, and the quick, darting manner of those who lived on their wits in a harsh land. He could spot things from a great distance – she had noticed him doing it when they were out in the bush. He could see a bird on a branch of an acacia tree when others could barely see the tree, and he could make out the light brown smudge of a nervous impala where others would think there was just grass and thorn bushes and sand.

'You could be a great tracker,' Mr J. L. B. Matekoni said to him once. 'You have that gift from your people.'

But Puso had turned away and said nothing. He is ashamed, thought Mr J. L. B. Matekoni; he is ashamed of what he is. He had tried to talk to him about it, but Puso had simply run away, out into the garden.

'What do we do, Mma Ramotswe?' asked Mr J. L. B. Matekoni. 'What do we say to him? Can you . . .'

'I'll try,' she said.

And she did, having waited for her moment, which came when she was sitting with Puso in her tiny white van. She was driving to Mochudi and he had come to keep her company, and she brought up the subject of his past.

'We took you and Motholeli in because we loved you,' she said. 'You know that, don't you?'

He looked down at his hands, folded on his lap in front of him. His voice was small when he replied. 'Yes. I know that.'

'And the only reason why you needed a new home was because your mother was late. She would have kept you if she had not become late. You know that, too?'

This time there was not even a murmur. She persisted, though. 'You can be proud of your mummy, you know, and of your daddy. The two peoples of this country. You are lucky to belong to both of them.'

He reached for the door handle, suddenly and without warning. He was so quick that she hardly saw it happen before the door was open and the wind was rushing in. Outside, the side of the road was a flash; the dusty brown of the verge, the black of the tar. She shouted out in alarm, and reached for him with one hand, her other hand remaining on the wheel, but slipping. At the same time, she braked sharply, sending the tiny white van sliding off the road. Puso, jolted forward by the braking motion, fell against the dashboard. He struggled to free himself from Mma Ramotswe's grip, but she held him tightly. He cried out.

For a few moments after the van had come to a halt, there was complete silence. The engine had stalled and there was just that odd, irregular ticking noise that comes from hot machinery, a settling down, a contracting of overheated parts.

'Are you all right?'

He did not answer her question, but sobbed. He turned his head away.

'You cannot jump out of a car,' stuttered Mma Ramotswe. The shock of what had happened had hit her, and she felt herself trembling.

Puso opened his eyes and looked at her briefly, as if to take her in for the first time. Then his gaze slid away. 'I don't want to be . . . that,' he said. 'I don't want to.'

Her heart went out to him. She reached forward and tried to hug him to her, but he wriggled out of her embrace.

'There is nothing wrong . . . nothing wrong with being what you are, Puso! Nothing.' She paused. The boy was still sobbing, his hands over his face, his frame shaking. She bent down to draw him close, overcoming his resistance, holding him to her. She had held her own child, had hugged the tiny figure, all those years ago, during those brief few hours of motherhood; and since then she had hardly done it. Now she did. It was an embrace that drew on the love which had somehow been stifled when she lost her child; drew on those wells of affection and feeling. Had she failed this little boy? Of course she had, and the realisation of this was painful to her. Why had she not given him the love that he so very much needed and that she, in turn, needed to give?

It was an effort for her not to cry too. But she could not cry, because she had to tell him something, and she could not talk and weep at the same time. 'Puso, I haven't spoken to you about this, and I'm sorry. I didn't think about it. I just didn't. Don't be cross with Mummy for that. Don't be cross with me.'

She stopped herself. She had said it. She had called herself his mother. She had not done that before; she had been Mma Ramotswe to the children, just as she was Mma Ramotswe to Mr J. L. B. Matekoni. She had not wanted to be their mother because she had been a mother, once, and was no longer. But that was wrong, so wrong. Of course she was a mother. We could all be a mother, all of us; even a man could be a mother.

Puso was looking at her. He began to say something, but did not; instead his eyes seemed to open wider and he stared at her in wonderment.

'Yes,' she said. 'You mustn't be cross with your mummy. I should have talked to you about these things that some people say. Unkind things about Masarwa. They're not true, you know. We are all the same. All the same people. Bushmen, San, whatever you want to call them, and us, Batswana. White people too. Everybody. Inside us, we are exactly the same. You know that, don't you? And we all come from the same mother, a long, long time ago, right here in Africa, up in East Africa somewhere. There was a lady who had some children, and they were the ancestors of every one of us, even of people who do not live in Africa. We are all the sons and daughters of that lady.'

He had stopped crying. His hand was resting on her wrist,

lightly, but she felt the warmth. She looked down at the miracle, the sheer miracle of human flesh, so vulnerable, so valuable.

'Better now?' It was not a good idea, she thought, to talk about these things at too great length. A few words were all that was needed.

He nodded, and she eased herself back into her seat and started the engine again. He reached for the handle of the passenger door and closed it.

'What was that lady's name?' he asked, as they continued their journey.

'Which lady?'

'That lady who had the children. The one in East Africa.'

She laughed. 'They didn't have names in those days, Puso. It was a long, long time ago. Long before Botswana.'

He looked disappointed. 'Makutsi, maybe.'

Mma Ramotswe bit her lip, suppressing a smile. For a moment she imagined an early woman, hirsute, half standing, half crouching, but wearing a large pair of glasses, like Mma Makutsi's. She took a hand off the wheel and reached out to touch him gently on the shoulder. Then he took her hand and held it briefly, before she put it back on the wheel so that the tiny white van might not go off the road again.

'Or maybe she was called Mma Ramotswe,' Puso said.

Now, sitting with Mr J. L. B. Matekoni on the verandah, she looked out into the dark of her garden. The light from the three-quarters moon was enough to reveal the shape of the shrubs, the outline of the mopipi tree, the flat umbrella of the acacia at the far end of her plot. By day her garden tended to reproach her, her eye always being drawn to the places where more watering was needed to keep things from wilting, or to those where the plants had withered and died; at night the bare patches were obscured, and forgiven.

'I had a letter today,' she said.

Mr J. L. B. Matekoni inclined his head. 'A letter?'

'Not a nice one.'

She told him of the contents, and he listened in silence. His voice was grave when he spoke. 'That is just what I have been worried about, Mma Ramotswe. It's what I've been fearing for a long time. Right from the beginning.'

'You've been worried that I would receive a letter like that?'

He shook his head. 'No. No. I have been worried that sooner or later you would come up against some really wicked person – some dangerous person who would try to harm you. Now you have.'

She reached out to put a reassuring hand on his arm. She knew that he was given to fretting about all sorts of things: about the garage, about the apprentices, about the state of the world; and she knew, too, that this was exactly what Dr Moffat had warned about. When Mr J. L. B. Matekoni had recovered from his depressive illness, Dr Moffat had said that he should avoid too much anxiety. 'You can't take away all of life's cares,' the doctor had said. 'But you can at least make sure that he doesn't worry too much. If he worries too much, the illness could return.'

I should not have told him about the letter, she thought. There was no point in burdening him with it when there was nothing that he could do about it and it would simply prey on his mind. But it was too late now; she had told him the exact contents of the letter and she could hardly take it back. Or could she?

'You know what I think, Mr J. L. B. Matekoni?' she said. 'I think that it's probably a joke. It's the sort of letter schoolboys write. They think that it's funny.'

For a moment he seemed to weigh this possibility, but then he shook his head again, more vigorously this time. 'It is not a joke, Mma Ramotswe. Those words are not the words of a schoolboy. They are the words of a dangerous person. A maniac.'

She tried to be dismissive. 'I don't think such a person is dangerous! Ridiculous, maybe; not dangerous.'

But her levity had no effect. He was becoming animated now, emphasising his points with movements of his hands. 'It makes me even more sure,' he said. 'It makes me certain that you should give it up. Detective work is not for women. It is for men who can look after themselves.'

Mma Ramotswe looked out into the darkness. He spoke in this way, she knew, because he loved her, and was anxious about her safety. She had suspected from time to time that he did not want her to continue with the agency, but she had always ignored these suspicions. She felt that in the fullness of time he would get used to her profession and what it entailed; that he would accept her calling, even be proud of it, in the way in which a husband can be proud of a successful wife. But she knew that once Mr J. L. B. Matekoni got an idea in his head, then it could be difficult to dislodge it. And this notion, she thought, was one of those that would be difficult to move.

Chapter Four

An Uncle with an
Unsophisticated, Broken Nose

As Mma Ramotswe and Mr J. L. B. Matekoni conversed on their verandah that evening, Mr Phuti Radiphuti sat in the modest living room of his fiancée, Mma Grace Makutsi, waiting for her to serve his dinner. They were having their meal rather later than usual that evening, as they had been shopping together and had been distracted by a display of beds in the large furniture store at River Walk. Phuti Radiphuti had been surprised at the prices, which he thought were below cost, but Mma Makutsi had been taken by the headboards, which not only were covered in a deep red velvet but were heart-shaped into the bargain.

'These are very fine beds,' she observed, reaching out to feel the texture of the velvet headboard. 'A person would sleep very well in a bed like that. And there is a lot of room, too.'

It was a potentially indelicate reference, at least in its last part, to the fact that these beds would accommodate both husband and wife in comfort; the sort of reference which, if made by an engaged woman to her fiancé, might be interpreted as a hint. Phuti Radiphuti and Mma Makutsi did not live together, and both had their own bed. This was Phuti's doing, and indeed Mma Makutsi had been slightly concerned that he had not been more passionate, so far. But that would come, she thought, in the fullness of time, and in the meantime there were plenty of matters to attend to without worrying about such things. As Mma Ramotswe had once delicately pointed out to Mma Makutsi, far too many people were permanently miserable because they allowed love affairs and everything that went with such things to dominate their lives. It is only one thing, she said, that business between men and women, and there are many other more important things, including food.

If Mma Makutsi's remarks on the bed and its heart-shaped headboard might have been interpreted by Phuti Radiphuti as a reproach, or indeed as an encouragement, this was not the way in which he took them.

'It would fit very well in my house,' he said. 'When we are married, this would be a very good bed for our room. And remember – beds are the one thing we don't sell at the Double Comfort Furniture Shop.'

Mma Makutsi caught her breath. They had a firm date, or

rather a tentatively firm date, for the wedding, but they had yet to deal with anything quite as concrete as a bed. This was progress, and she tried very hard to conceal her excitement. 'You're right,' she said. 'And this velvet is very fine. Feel it.'

Phuti Radiphuti stretched out to run his fingers over the soft cloth. 'Very good,' he said. 'But I don't see how they can do this bed at this price. Where's their profit?' He paused, glancing at the price of a nearby set of chairs. 'A loss leader,' he said. 'That is what they are doing. It's an old trick.'

Mma Makutsi wondered whether she should suggest that he purchase the bed. She, of course, could not buy it herself, as she had very little money of her own. Her financial position had been immeasurably improved when she set up her small, part-time typing school for men, but that had now been abandoned and she was dependent on her salary from the No. 1 Ladies' Detective Agency. Even with Mma Ramotswe's generous rates of pay, that was not much; the agency barely made a profit and effectively relied on subventions from Mma Ramotswe's own purse – she still had her fine herd of cattle, which meant that she was comfortably off – and from Tlokweng Road Speedy Motors, in the form of rent-free premises.

Phuti Radiphuti was a kind man, and he was tactful in the exercise of his generosity. He had stopped short of giving Mma Makutsi an allowance, but he had taken on many of her expenses, paying grocery bills and giving her regular and frequent presents. Now he raised a hand to attract the attention of one of the assistants who had been hovering in the background.

'That is a very good bed, Rra,' said the assistant, sensing a sale. 'And you and your wife will like it. It suits you.'

Phuti Radiphuti appeared momentarily flustered. He began to stammer. 'I . . . I—'

'We are not yet married,' Mma Makutsi cut in. 'We are engaged now, but not yet married. That will happen soon.'

The assistant apologised fulsomely. He saw the ring on her finger, that ring with the dazzling Botswana diamond, her proudest possession, the symbol of the man who loved her, and of the country they both loved; such purity and light. 'I thought . . . You looked as if you were married, Mma. And soon you will be.'

'Quite soon,' said Mma Makutsi.

The assistant looked down at the floor.

'I will buy this bed,' said Phuti Radiphuti, recovering from his embarrassment. 'Yes, I will take it.'

The assistant's face broke into a smile. He made a little boxing feint in the air, narrowly missing Phuti Radiphuti in his exuberance. 'An excellent decision, Rra. It's a very good buy.' He took a notebook out of his pocket and began to take Phuti's details. The bed, he said, would be delivered the following day. And then, 'Will you be buying the headboard too, Rra?'

The unexpected question hung unanswered in the air. Mma Makutsi glanced at Phuti Radiphuti, who was looking in a worried way at the price tag on the bed. 'But it says . . .' he began.

The assistant bent down to point to the wording at the bottom of the tag. 'You'll see, Rra,' he said, 'that the headboard is excluded. You see here. It says, "headboard excluded". The headboard is twelve hundred pula, Rra.' He paused. 'That is a very big bargain, I think.'

Mma Makutsi thought. Twelve hundred pula was almost her monthly salary; for many people it was more than that. Her cousins up in Bobonong, where there was little work, would have to save for months, a year perhaps, to accumulate such an amount.

Phuti hesitated. 'You . . . You sh . . . should . . .' He was beginning to stammer. Mma Makutsi frowned at the assistant. It was his fault that this misunderstanding had arisen – he should have made it clear at the outset that the bed and the headboard were separate items. And now Phuti's stammer was starting again, which was frustrating for her, after all the efforts she had made to help him overcome it. Perhaps she should ask to speak to the manager and give him a piece of her mind about the need to make terms and conditions clear to customers. In her business practice course at the Botswana Secretarial College they had stressed that one should never try to mislead the customer. And indeed Clovis Andersen, whose book Mma Ramotswe was always going on about, said much the same thing about telling the truth to clients. *Never put anything in small print and then spring it on the client. That breaks trust.*

'That breaks trust,' she muttered.

The assistant only half heard her. 'What was that, Mma?'

Phuti cleared his throat. 'I'll take the headboard too,' he said. The stammer had gone, replaced by a note of resignation in his voice.

'We'll deliver them both tomorrow,' said the assistant. 'To your address, Rra?'

Phuti turned to Mma Makutsi. 'It can go to your house first, Grace,' he said. 'You can enjoy sleeping in it until we move it to my house after the wedding.'

Mma Makutsi accepted demurely. She gave the address to the assistant, who wrote it down in his notebook. So much had changed in her life since she had become engaged to Phuti. Now, with the arrangements being made for the delivery of the bed, it seemed to her that a further, tangible improvement was about to be achieved. This bed, with its elaborate headboard, would have been an impossible self-indulgence in her earlier state. Phuti had made the decision to purchase the bed as if the expense were something that one would hardly notice, and yet it had cost so much. She wondered if that was what it would be like to have buying power – not having to worry about what one had to pay, but deciding whether or not to buy something purely on the basis of whether one wanted it. And would that apply, she asked herself, to shoes? For a moment she imagined the shoes she might have – a cupboard full of new shoes, all set out on racks. She would wear a different colour each day, depending on her mood, and perhaps take a spare pair along with her to work so that she could change them as the spirit moved her. She closed her eyes at the thought.

So that's what you think of us, Boss! Too grand for us – after all we've done for you! The voice of her shoes, her green shoes with sky-blue linings, was filled with reproach, and her eyes popped open. She looked away, ashamed at her greed.

She would have to be careful. It was all very well becoming Mrs Phuti Radiphuti, wife of the proprietor of the Double Comfort Furniture Shop, but one should not forget where it was that one had come from; although, if one did, there were always one's shoes to remind one.

Curiously enough, while Mma Makutsi prepared Phuti Radiphuti's dinner that evening, happily anticipating the arrival of the new bed the following morning, Mr J. L. B. Matekoni and Mma Ramotswe, comfortably seated on their verandah, were talking about her. Although their conversation did not have anything to do – directly – with the bed in question, none the less it did concern an intimate problem arising from Mma Makutsi's engagement.

'Mma Makutsi spoke to me about her engagement this morning,' said Mma Ramotswe. 'We were having tea . . .'

Mr J. L. B. Matekoni smiled. They were always having tea, as far as he could work out. There was the first cup, served shortly after they arrived in the office in the morning, and then there was the ten o'clock cup, which was sometimes taken at nine thirty in the hot weather. That was followed by the tea which was brewed at eleven thirty (the mid-morning tea), and of course there was tea immediately after lunch and again at three in the afternoon. He thought it was a good thing that the red bush tea contained no caffeine, or Mma Ramotswe would surely find it difficult to get to sleep at night, with all that caffeine in her system. Yet Mma Makutsi drank ordinary tea, which had ample quantities of caffeine in it, he believed;

indeed he thought that this might explain why she was sometimes so tetchy with the apprentices, especially with Charlie.
Mind you, anybody might be forgiven for being irritated by
Charlie, with his constant boasting and that endless silly chat-
ter about girls; even one with no caffeine at all in his system
could find himself snapping at such a young man.

'Her engagement? That is a long story.' He laughed, but
stopped himself quickly. His own engagement had not been
exactly brief. It had lasted for some years and had only been
brought to a successful conclusion when Mma Potokwani
had somehow managed to stand with Mma Ramotswe before
that improvised altar on the orphan farm. He did not regret
that day for one moment, and the memory of it was unquestion-
ably a warm one; but the length of the preceding engagement perhaps precluded his passing comment on the length
of time for which Mma Makutsi and Phuti Radiphuti were
engaged.

So he said, 'Not that engagements should not be a long
story, Mma. It is better, is it not, to be sure of the person you
are marrying before you marry. That is what I have always
thought.'

Mma Ramotswe suppressed a smile, remembering how she
had almost resigned herself to a date's never being set for their
wedding. If Mma Potokwani owed Mr J. L. B. Matekoni a
great deal for all that he had done for her by way of fixing
things, then she herself owed a heavy debt of gratitude to the
orphan farm matron for managing to cajole her husband into
marriage. But that, she thought, was what so much of life was

like: we allowed one another something for some service or favour, sometimes for something done a long time ago, even before our birth; debts to parents, debts to ancestors.

'No,' Mma Ramotswe agreed. 'One does not want to marry too quickly. Nor too slowly, perhaps . . . But Mma Makutsi did not say that Phuti Radiphuti was refusing to name a day. He has done that now.'

Mr J. L. B. Matekoni looked puzzled. 'So what can the problem be? If they have decided on a day—'

'The day is not the issue. It is the *bogadi*.'

'Ah!' Mr J. L. B. Matekoni understood now. *Bogadi*, or *lobola*, was the dowry that the Radiphutis would have to pay to Mma Makutsi's people. This would have to be negotiated before the formal agreement between the families would bring the marriage into existence.

After Mr J. L. B. Matekoni had said Ah, there was a brief silence. Then he continued, firstly by saying Ah again, and then, 'Eight cattle. Maybe nine.'

Mma Ramotswe appeared to consider this for a moment. 'Some people might say six head of cattle for a lady like Mma Makutsi. I am not saying that she is not pretty – I think she is – but—'

'It depends on the light,' said Mr J. L. B. Matekoni. He spoke seriously, and did not intend his remark to be barbed: it really did depend on the light, he thought. Strong sunlight, especially when it came from such an angle that it glinted off Mma Makutsi's glasses, was not flattering. But when the light was weaker – at dusk, for example – then her high cheekbones stood out in an interesting way. He had noticed that and had even once mentioned the fact to Mma Ramotswe, who had said nothing, but had looked at him in a way which suggested that he should return to working on his cars. Women did not like men to discuss the appearance of other women, although they liked to do so themselves, he had noticed; and no woman would object to a man's discussing her own appearance, in complimentary terms of course.

Mma Ramotswe was loyal. 'Mma Makutsi is pretty in every light, I think. When I said "but" I was about to say that there are some people who think that her glasses are too big.'

'I am one of those,' said Mr J. L. B. Matekoni. 'Are big glasses more powerful than small glasses? I do not think so: it is what is in the glass that counts, not how much glass there is.' He paused. 'But her eyes are quite big, aren't they? Have you seen them, Mma Ramotswe? They are big, like the eyes of a kudu.'

Mma Ramotswe felt uncomfortable at the direction the conversation was taking. She had not intended that they should get into such a detailed discussion of Mma Makutsi's appearance, and she decided that it was time to return to the subject of the dowry.

'This *bogadi* business,' she said. 'I have never been sure about it, Mr J. L. B. Matekoni.'

Mr J. L. B. Matekoni had paid ten cattle for Mma Ramotswe. Was she now offering to give them back? 'Those ten cattle I paid,' he began. 'Ten good cattle. Fat ones . . .'

The cattle had certainly been large, sweet-smelling beasts

53

who had been specially fed on bales of lucerne bought at some expense from over the border; they had grown fat and their coats had shone with health. They were a worthy tribute to Mma Ramotswe and although three had been taken by one of her uncles, and another had been slaughtered for the marriage feast of one of her cousins, those that remained were out at her cattle post and by all accounts doing well.

She made it clear that it was not those cattle she was talking about. The negotiations that had preceded their marriage had been model ones, with her family readily agreeing to what was proposed by the aged uncle who had acted for Mr J. L. B. Matekoni. No, that was not the sort of case that concerned her; she was worried about those cases where the husband had great difficulty in finding the means to pay the bride price. People got themselves into debt; they spent money which should have been spent on other things. But most of all she thought that the whole idea made women seem like property – *things* that could be bought.

'Would it not be better if a man did not have to pay for his wife?' she asked Mr J. L. B. Matekoni. 'I am not one to disturb old customs unnecessarily, but wouldn't it be better?'

Rather to her surprise, Mr J. L. B. Matekoni was quick to agree. 'Yes. It would be better. You pay for a car, you do not pay for a wife.'

Mma Ramotswe looked at him with admiration. 'That is a very modern view, Mr J. L. B. Matekoni,' she said, almost adding 'for a man', but not doing so. Men could be modern, too, she reminded herself.

Mr J. L. B. Matekoni now added something instead. 'Of course, you cannot take a wife back as you can take a car back. There is a difference there.'

Mma Ramotswe frowned. She was not sure why he had said this or what it meant, but she decided not to seek clarification. Mr J. L. B. Matekoni generally meant well, and was respectful of women – unlike the apprentices.

'What's worrying me,' she said, 'is the negotiations. Did you hear that Mma Makutsi's uncle has been down in Gaborone?'

Mr J. L. B. Matekoni had not heard this. 'Nobody tells me about these matters,' he said. 'I did not know that.'

'Well, he has been. He is a very odd-looking man with a broken nose. I caught a glimpse of him when I dropped her off after work one afternoon. He came to the gate.'

'There are some strange people up there,' said Mr J. L. B. Matekoni. 'Bobonong, isn't it?'

Mma Ramotswe nodded. 'That is where they are from. Not all people from up there are like that, but sometimes . . .'

'I wonder how his nose was broken,' mused Mr J.L.B. Matekoni. 'I knew a mechanic once who had a car door slammed on his nose. It was a very bad thing to happen.'

Mma Ramotswe drew in her breath sharply. 'On his *nose*?'

'Yes,' said Mr J. L. B. Matekoni. 'It was very sore, I think.'

Mma Ramotswe was puzzled. 'But how did it happen? Why was his nose in the way?' She could understand how fingers got slammed in car doors, but it would be difficult, she thought, to get one's nose in the wrong place.

'He was leaning into the car,' said Mr J. L. B. Matekoni. 'And I think that his nose was quite a long one.'

For a moment neither of them spoke. There were many dangers in this world, and the longer one journeyed through life the more one understood how varied these dangers were. That, thought Mma Ramotswe, was why one worried more and more about others: one could imagine the manifold disasters that might befall them. And she did not want anything unpleasant to happen to others; Mma Ramotswe wished ill on nobody. In particular, she would not wish that any man, no matter how long his nose, should suffer indignity and pain on that account.

She brought the conversation back to Mma Makutsi's uncle. 'He is a greedy man, I fear. He has asked for too much.'

Mr J. L. B. Matekoni sighed. 'That is exactly what an uncle should *not* do,' he said. 'It makes everything very complicated.'

'Exactly.' Mma Ramotswe paused. 'You said eight cattle for Mma Makutsi?'

'That would be about right,' said Mr J. L. B. Matekoni. 'She is a competent lady. She is educated. And the Radiphuti family can easily afford eight cattle.'

'All of that is true,' said Mma Ramotswe. 'But in this case, do you know what he asked for?'

Mr J. L. B. Matekoni tried to put himself in the position of the uncle from Bobonong. Such a man would be very impressed by the Double Comfort Furniture Shop. He would not know about overheads and bad debts and all the things that sapped the profits of a business. In the mind of an uncle from Bobonong, an uncle with an unsophisticated, broken nose, the owner of a large store would be unimaginably wealthy, and have many cattle. 'Twenty?' he ventured. Twenty would be an outrageously large *bogadi*; far more than Mma Makutsi was worth.

'No,' said Mma Ramotswe. And then, with the air of one disclosing a scandalous fact, 'Ninety-seven.'

Mr J. L. B. Matekoni's eyes revealed his surprise. But then he remembered, and he began to smile. A wily uncle indeed; one who had absorbed the salient facts of family history.

'Because . . .' he began.

'Yes,' said Mma Ramotswe. 'Because.'

Then they both laughed.

Chapter Five

Could One Rend
the Heart in Two?

How, Mma Ramotswe asked herself, do you put together the story of a life when you don't know the very beginning – who your parents were?

She looked past Mma Makutsi's unattended desk, out through the window and onto the branches of the acacia tree outside. It was the morning following the conversation with Mr J. L. B. Matekoni in which they had discussed the absurd demands of Mma Makutsi's uncle, and she was by herself. Mma Makutsi would be in the office that morning, but only later on: she had arranged with Mma Ramotswe to come in at eleven, after the delivery van had delivered her new bed.

Could One Rend the Heart in Two?

'A new bed?' Mma Ramotswe had asked. 'That is very good.'

She spoke without thinking why it should be particularly good to receive a new bed, but a moment's subsequent thought justified the comment. Many people, she felt, did not have a good night's sleep, and this was often because they did not have a good bed. And if you did not have a good night's sleep, it showed in the way you behaved towards others. Some of her clients, she thought – the irritable or irascible ones – probably did not have a good bed, and would have been much improved by a night or two in a more comfortable place; not that she could tell them that, of course.

She imagined the scene. 'I think I know the answer to your problem, Rra,' she would say. 'It is in your bed. That is where the answer lies.'

Such advice would not be well received, and could well be misinterpreted. The client might take it as a disparaging reference to a wife or husband, for example, and it could be awkward explaining that the solution lay in the mattress rather than in any person *upon* the mattress. Mind you, that was often the case too, she suspected, but she could not say that either.

Mma Ramotswe sighed and took a sip from her cup of bush tea. She had been obliged to make the tea herself, in the absence of Mma Makutsi, and this brought home to her the implications of Mma Makutsi's marriage, if it ever took place. Her assistant had spontaneously assured her that becoming Mrs Phuti Radiphuti would make no difference to her career, and that she had every intention of continuing to work as an associate detective, but Mma Ramotswe wondered about this. She did not doubt the sincerity of Mma Makutsi's assurance – Mma Makutsi would never lie to her – but she wondered whether the distractions involved in being married to a man with a large furniture store would simply prove too much for her assistant. And if that were to be the case, then who would make the tea in the agency? And who would collect the mail, and do the filing, and answer the telephone? And who would go out to buy doughnuts from the Lucky Chance Tuck Shop round the corner on Friday mornings, when they treated themselves?

There were so many respects in which Mma Makutsi would be missed – not only in those practical ways, but in ways connected with the moral support she gave Mma Ramotswe and in the inspiration which so often flowed from their casual discussion of a troubling case. Mma Makutsi tackled problems from a slightly different angle than did Mma Ramotswe, and asked slightly different questions. That perspective often led to a solution, and cut short the time which Mma Ramotswe would otherwise have spent on a case. It would be sorely missed, as would the tea and the doughnuts, and all the rest.

Now, for instance, in the absence of Mma Makutsi, Mma Ramotswe was having to work out for herself how she might approach the case of Mma Sebina, with her hidden past and her unknown relatives. If Mma Makutsi had been there, she might well have said something which would trigger a productive line of inquiry. But she was not, and there was no point in speculating what she might have said. Or was there?

Mma Ramotswe closed her eyes for a moment and imagined her assistant at her desk.

'Now then, Mma Makutsi,' she muttered. 'What do we have here? We have Mma Sebina, who now knows that her mother was not her mother and her father was not her father. So that means that—'

'Wait a moment, Mma,' said the imaginary Mma Makutsi. 'All you know, Mma Ramotswe, is that the late mother told somebody that she was not the mother. Does that mean we can say for sure that Mma Sebina was not the daughter of that lady? Does it really mean that, Mma?'

It was an unexpected question, but it made Mma Ramotswe pause. She had often taken Mma Makutsi to task for assuming things too readily, and now here was her assistant accusing her of exactly the same thing.

Her eyes still firmly shut, Mma Ramotswe spread her hands in a gesture of acceptance. 'You're quite right, Mma,' she said. 'It is possible that the mother – that is, the lady who was known as the mother – was really the mother after all and was lying when she told that other lady that she was not. That is possible, I think.'

Mma Makutsi shook her head. 'No, Mma,' she said. 'You have misunderstood me. Perhaps the lady who said that the other lady said that thing – perhaps *that* is the lady who was making up the story. That is what I meant.'

Mma Ramotswe smiled. 'Why, of course! A real mother would not lie about such a matter, particularly when she was very ill and would shortly be called to account for all her lies, if she had any. She would not lie then, even if she had been a liar before, would she?'

'Excuse me, Mma.' It was not Mma Makutsi's voice, but another voice altogether, and Mma Ramotswe opened her eyes with a start. Mr Polopetsi, the general assistant at the garage and their occasional helper in the agency, was standing in the door, framed by the morning sunlight, an empty mug in his hand.

'I heard you talking,' he said. 'And I knocked. Like this. Knock, knock. But you did not hear me. You were busy talking to . . . to . . .'

His embarrassment was evident, and Mma Ramotswe, although herself embarrassed to have been found talking to herself, sought to reassure him.

'To Mma Makutsi,' she said. 'I was talking to Mma Makutsi, Rra.'

Mr Polopetsi glanced at Mma Makutsi's empty desk. 'I see.'

Mma Ramotswe laughed. 'No, she is not there, Mr Polopetsi. There is no Mma Makutsi. I was thinking of what I would say to her, you see. I was imagining that we were talking to one another. But she is not there . . . as you can see,' she ended lamely.

'No, she is not there,' said Mr Polopetsi, advancing towards the teapot. 'That is correct. She is not there, Mma.'

'Exactly,' said Mma Ramotswe. 'But I closed my eyes to imagine that she was there, because I needed to know what she would think about something.'

'I see,' said Mr Polopetsi, as he filled his mug with tea from

Mma Ramotswe's teapot. 'But who is this lady who has no mother?'

Mma Ramotswe looked at the man standing before her and watched him take a sip of his freshly poured tea. There was something vulnerable about Mr Polopetsi that always made her feel slightly sorry for him. But she liked him, and indeed had liked him from the time when they had first met in those inauspicious circumstances almost two years previously. Mma Ramotswe had inadvertently knocked him off his bicycle when she was driving to Tlokweng in her tiny white van. She had picked him up, driven him home, and arranged for the repair of the buckled bicycle wheel. After that, she had persuaded Mr J. L. B. Matekoni to take him on as an assistant in the garage – a role in which he had quickly showed his worth. Since then, if there was not enough work for him in the garage, he had helped in the agency, not on major cases – if any of their cases could be called major, which was doubtful – but on small inquiries, particularly on those which required a man rather than a woman. Mma Ramotswe could not go into a bar, for example, without attracting attention, whereas a slight man like Mr Polopetsi could slip into a bar virtually unnoticed.

'The lady without a mother is a new client,' she explained. 'Her name is Mma Sebina. She is an orphan.'

'We are all orphans,' said Mr Polopetsi. 'I am an orphan. And you, too, Mma Ramotswe, you are an orphan.'

Mma Ramotswe smiled. 'Yes, I suppose we are. But it is different for us. We know who our late parents were. This lady is not sure who they were and that is what she wants me to find out.'

Mr Polopetsi blew across the rim of his mug to cool the tea. A small wisp of steam was caught in a beam of sunlight from the window, and vanished. 'I suppose that is something we all want to know,' he said reflectively. 'Have you noticed how people seem very interested in these family things when they get older? Sixty is when it starts. That is when they really want to know who were their parents' parents and the parents of those ones before them. Right, right back to Chief Sechele's days.' He paused, sipping at his tea. Mma Ramotswe noticed how he puckered his lips when he sipped; like a bushbuck drinking from the water, she thought. But perhaps we were all like some animal or another, not just Mr Polopetsi, who looked so much like one of those timid creatures one saw in the bush at the side of the road, ready to dart off into the undergrowth. And of course she had run him down, just as people sometimes ran small antelope down on the bush roads.

'Mind you,' continued Mr Polopetsi, 'mind you, I can understand why people want to find these things out. If you'll be joining the ancestors, it's useful to know who the ancestors are before you meet them.'

Mma Ramotswe stared at him in surprise. Mr Polopetsi was a modern man, who had been a pharmacy assistant. He knew about chemicals and the like, and here he was talking about the ancestors. Usually if educated people believed in such things they were discreet about it. It was not fashionable to go on about the ancestors in public.

She decided to ask him directly. 'Do you think that it's true, Rra? Do you think that the ancestors are up there, waiting for us?'

Mr Polopetsi looked into his mug. Mma Ramotswe watched him and suppressed an irreverent thought. It was as if he was searching for ancestors there, in his mug of bush tea.

'The ancestors,' he began portentously. 'The ancestors . . .'

She waited for him to continue, but he was silent, as if defeated by the sheer weight of the topic, or of the ancestors perhaps.

'I think that they are with us,' she said. 'They are all around us. What they have done. Their voices. The memories they have left us. All of that is there.'

He looked up sharply, with the air of one to whom a major discovery is announced, an annunciation. 'That is a very good way of putting it,' he said. 'That is very good, Mma. Yes, indeed. That is how I shall think of it in the future.'

Mma Ramotswe smiled modestly. She was not sure if she had said anything very significant; in fact, she felt that what she had said did not really address the question of whether the ancestors were there or not, in the sense that being there meant actual existence. She had not answered that question directly; in fact, she had not answered it at all. But if what she had said to Mr Polopetsi was at all helpful, then she was pleased with that.

'But getting back to this Mma Sebina and her problems,' she said. 'She thinks that she was looked after by a lady who was not her mother. Now that lady is late and she says that there are no relatives she knows of on that side. That is very unusual, of course, as everybody has relatives. But apparently that lady and her husband had none, or none that they ever mentioned.'

'So now she is alone?'

'It looks like it.'

For a few moments they were both silent as they contemplated Mma Sebina's situation. In a country like Botswana, it was almost inconceivable to be completely alone, to have no family. What would it be like to have nobody? Such loneliness was hard to imagine.

Mr Polopetsi took a final sip of his tea and put his mug down on Mma Makutsi's desk. He would not have dared to do that if Mma Makutsi had been there, thought Mma Ramotswe, but why should he not avail himself of the nearest surface? It was not as if Mma Makutsi *owned* her desk; it belongs to me, thought Mma Ramotswe, and I could give him permission if I wanted to.

'You must find people for her,' said Mr Polopetsi. 'That is what you must do, Mma Ramotswe.'

Mma Ramotswe sighed. 'I know that, Rra. That is what she asked me to do. That is why she came here.'

He nodded encouragingly.

'But I'm not sure how I should begin,' she went on. 'The person who must know where she comes from is the lady who acted as mother. But how do you ask a question of someone who is late? Especially if that person had no relatives herself?'

Mr Polopetsi looked out of the window. 'But she must have

had somebody, even if she didn't know. She must have come from somewhere. Somebody must know something about her.'

That was true, conceded Mma Ramotswe. But did it take them any further in their inquiry? They were not trying to trace the relatives of that woman herself; it was Mma Sebina's relatives they were looking for.

Mr Polopetsi agreed. 'But if we find people who knew something about her – the late mother who wasn't the real mother – then we could find out whether she ever said anything about her daughter. We could find out if anybody remembered the baby arriving. After all, if a baby suddenly comes to a house and the lady of that house has not been seen to be pregnant, people will ask: where is this baby from? That is what they will ask. Babies do not come out of thin air.'

That was true, thought Mma Ramotswe. But then she thought that perhaps it was not. There were plenty of people who came out of thin air; they turned up in our lives and we accepted them without question. Even you, Mr Polopetsi, she thought, even you. You came into our lives out of thin air. I did not see you before I knocked you down. You came out of thin air, which is exactly how I put it to Mr J. L. B. Matekoni when he asked me how I had managed to knock you off your bicycle. 'He came out of thin air,' I said.

She did not say anything of that. Instead, she looked at her watch and said, 'I think you should work on this case with me, Rra. If the garage is not very busy Mr J. L. B. Matekoni will not mind.'

Mr Polopetsi glanced through the door into the garage workshop beyond. 'There is not much going on through there,' he said. 'If you give me just an hour or so I shall finish doing one or two things through there. Then I shall be ready.'

Mma Ramotswe agreed. He could have the hour in the garage, and then they would go off to the small village south of Gaborone where Mma Sebina had started her life's journey, or where she *might* have started it. While Mr Polopetsi busied himself with his remaining garage chores, Mma Ramotswe tackled the morning's filing, a task normally performed by Mma Makutsi. She could have left it, of course, for Mma Makutsi to do when she came in later, but she had nothing else to do and it would be interesting, she decided, to see whether she would be able to adapt herself to the system which Mma Makutsi used; she would have to do this if the new Mrs Phuti Radiphuti ended up working in the Double Comfort Furniture Shop rather than in the No. 1 Ladies' Detective Agency, as was perfectly possible.

She got up and walked over to the battered filing cabinet that stood halfway between her desk and the desk occupied by Mma Makutsi. They would have to replace that cabinet, which had been acquired right at the beginning, when the No. 1 Ladies' Detective Agency was first set up. They had been in her first office then, that small breeze-block building in the shadow of Kgale Hill, where those insolent chickens had wandered in and pecked at the floor around one's toes; such silly creatures, with their tattered combs and their scruffy leg feathers like tiny pantaloons. The filing cabinet had been virtually the first piece of office furniture then; there had not even been a proper desk for Mma Makutsi, who had been obliged to make do with a table that had been used for making tea on in the Water Affairs office but had been sold as surplus to requirements. They had entertained such high hopes, then, for their little agency, and had so quickly abandoned those hopes when no clients turned up for week after week. And the filing cabinet then was empty, quite empty, as they had received no letters from anybody and had no papers to file. Eventually, in desperation, Mma Makutsi had filed a tattered circular which somebody had slipped through the door. That circular, Mma Makutsi had told her the other day, was still there, as a reminder of how slow things had been and of how great things may come from moments of nothingness. Perhaps we should all do that, thought Mma Ramotswe. Perhaps we should all keep a few things, a few mementoes, to remind us of what we used to be, just in case we forgot. If I ever became really rich, she thought, rich enough to own a Mercedes-Benz, what would I keep of the tiny white van to remind me of what I used to drive? The steering wheel – perhaps inserted into the Mercedes-Benz by Mr J. L. B. Matekoni in place of its grand new wheel, just to remind me? She smiled at the thought.

She pulled on the handle of the filing cabinet's top drawer. It was stiff and would not budge. She pulled at it again, this time lifting it slightly; she remembered that this drawer was a difficult one and could get stuck. There was still no movement and so she tried the drawer below, the one which Mma Makutsi had labelled *Concluded Affairs*. It was such a strange label for a filing drawer; as if the drawer contained the love letters, the keepsakes, of a crowded personal past. If she managed to get *Concluded Affairs* to open, then perhaps its upstairs neighbour, *Current Investigations*, might be more obliging.

When *Concluded Affairs* stubbornly refused to open, it occurred to Mma Ramotswe that the filing cabinet was locked. This conclusion brought mixed emotions. On the one hand, it said a great deal for Mma Makutsi's attentiveness and sense of responsibility that she should lock a filing cabinet which contained a great deal of highly personal information. There were letters from clients in those drawers, letters in which they revealed some of their most intimate concerns – suspicions of adultery, thoughts about the character of others, stories of intrigue and bad behaviour. All of that would have been a godsend to a blackmailer, or even a gossip. So it was a wise precaution to lock it all away.

But then she thought: it would have been helpful if Mma Makutsi had told her that the filing cabinet was locked and, moreover, where the key was kept. What if Mma Makutsi were out of the office – as she was now – and Mma Ramotswe needed to make a sudden reference to a current investigation or even a concluded affair? What then?

She turned round and looked down at Mma Makutsi's desk. There were two drawers in this desk. Mma Ramotswe knew that one of these was used for the storage of such things as rubber bands and paper clips. The other was, she thought, a more personal drawer, into which Mma Makutsi tucked things such as those lace handkerchiefs for which she had a particular fondness. If the key was stored anywhere in the office, then that, she thought, would be where it was.

Feeling slightly furtive, Mma Ramotswe moved to the other side of the desk and gingerly opened the top drawer. It, at least, was unlocked, and slid open easily. She looked down. There was a bottle of aspirin – Mma Makutsi had a tendency to headaches at the height of the hot season – a folded handkerchief, a metal bottle opener with a picture of Table Mountain etched on the shaft, and a photograph. She reached down and picked up the photograph. It was Phuti Radiphuti, standing in front of a door, his arms folded, self-consciously posed. He looked so serious, so self-important, that Mma Ramotswe could not help but smile. And then she laughed; not in an unkindly way, because she liked Phuti, and she was not a person to laugh at another. It was just so odd, that position of his: what on earth could have possessed Phuti Radiphuti to strike such a ridiculous pose?

Then Mma Makutsi came into the room. She was carrying a brown paper bag in her hands: doughnuts. The fat from the doughnuts had seeped through the paper; round tracings of grease. When she saw Mma Ramotswe with the photograph of Phuti Radiphuti, she stood quite still, her eyes moving from the photograph to Mma Ramotswe's face, caught in its smile, and then back down to the photograph.

The doughnuts, of course, were a sign: doughnuts on Friday were normal, but doughnuts purchased on any other day meant that Mma Makutsi felt that she needed cheering up.

And that particular morning, cheering up was exactly what was required.

It was not that the day had started badly; it had not. Mma Makutsi had awoken in a state of excitement, as one does when one has been vouchsafed a satisfying dream or when the day ahead brings the prospect of some numinous event. As she stretched out in her rather small and uncomfortable bed – the lumps in her mattress had always been in the wrong place – she reflected on how that coming night she would be sleeping in the unimaginable luxury of the new bed. She looked at her watch and saw that it was time to get up, which was not a chore, not that morning. She would have a lukewarm shower – the heating system never managed more than a few degrees of boost above the prevailing temperature – and then she would prepare her breakfast. They had promised to deliver the new bed early, and she wanted to be ready for them when they came. Delivery men could be awkward about moving existing furniture and they would need at least a cup of strong tea and a sandwich before agreeing to stack her old bed and mattress against the back wall. The food would be ready when they arrived and then . . . she closed her eyes in bliss.

The men came at the appointed time; one man driving a top-heavy blue van, the other in the passenger seat counting out the plot numbers as they made their way down Mma Makutsi's dusty road. When she saw them, she went out to the gate and waved them down.

'I am the person,' she called out. 'It is my bed.'

The van came to a halt and the men got out. Civilities were

exchanged. Had she slept well? She had. Had they? They too had slept well. Then the opening of the back door of the van and the manoeuvring out of a great, plastic-wrapped object. There was a wind, a small wind blowing tiny eddies of dust, and it caught the edge of the transparent plastic wrapping and made it flap. I am filled with pride, Mma Makutsi thought. I am filled with pride.

The men carried the bed through the gate and into Mma Makutsi's yard, where they propped it up against the front wall. The large object seemed to dwarf the house; a big bed for a small house, thought Mma Makutsi.

'Very beautiful,' said the driver as he began to cut at the plastic wrapping. 'One of the most beautiful beds in Botswana.'

'Yes,' said Mma Makutsi. 'That's why we chose it, Rra.'

The two men tugged at the last remaining shreds of plastic. The large velvet heart was now revealed, although it was not yet in position, but was tied to the base of the bed. With a deft movement, the men detached it and stacked it next to the base of the bed.

'There is a bed in there already,' said Mma Makutsi. 'I wondered if you could move it for me?'

The men glanced at one another. 'There is always another bed,' the driver's assistant said.

The driver frowned. 'We can help you, Mma. Don't worry.'

They went inside and Mma Makutsi showed them her bed. With the sheets and blankets taken off, it was a sad, dejected thing. The men, though, were businesslike; there was no time for emotion in the bed-moving business. It took them no more than a few minutes to unscrew the legs and manhandle the base out into the back yard. Then, dusting their hands, they returned to the new bed and began to carry it towards the door. Mma Makutsi watched in pride and pleasure. She would have to get new sheets, she decided, to do justice to this luxurious acquisition.

'This bed won't go through the door,' the driver said. 'Look, Mma. It is too big.'

Mma Makutsi gave a start. 'But it must fit, Rra,' she said. 'They wouldn't make a bed that won't fit.'

The driver laughed. 'Don't be too sure of that, Mma,' he said. 'I have seen many people buy furniture that is too big for their houses. We see that all the time, don't we?'

His assistant nodded. 'Remember those chairs, Boss? Remember those people who lived in that very small house and they bought those great big chairs?'

The driver laughed again. 'They were small people too,' he said. 'I can never understand why small people think they need big furniture.'

Mma Makutsi stepped forward to examine the bed. It stood, sideways on, against the door and was clearly a foot or so too large to fit in.

'The only way would be to take the roof off,' said the driver. 'I have seen that done before.'

'I cannot take the roof off,' snapped Mma Makutsi. 'I am only a tenant here. I cannot take the roof off.'

The driver shrugged. 'It is too late to take this bed back,' he said. 'We are under strict instructions: never bring anything back. I'm sorry about that, Mma.'

'Then please move the bed to the side there,' said Mma Makutsi. 'I will speak to my fiancé about it.'

They moved the new bed to the side of the house and put the old bed back. Then they began to take their leave. 'I'm sorry,' said the driver. 'It is a fine bed, but . . .' He made a gesture with his hands, a gesture that was somewhere between a denial of further responsibility and an indication of sympathy.

Mma Makutsi watched them leave. She was at a complete loss as to what to do. It was difficult to see what could be done to make the bed fit, short of sawing it in two and making a couple of single beds out of it – but what would happen to the heart? Could one rend the heart in two? One could not.

And it was at that point that the idea came to her: she would buy some doughnuts.

Chapter Six

A Chair in a Tree

It was a considerable relief for Mma Ramotswe when she eventually got out of the office with Mr Polopetsi and set off in her tiny white van. There had been the embarrassment of being found looking at a photograph of Phuti Radiphuti and smiling – just smiling, she insisted to Mma Makutsi.

'I was not laughing, Mma,' she insisted when she saw the look on her assistant's face. 'This is a very fine photograph. It's just that the person taking it has made him look so severe, with those folded arms. Like a judge.'

Mma Makutsi had reached out for the photograph and taken it from her. 'That is a private photograph, Mma,' she said in an injured tone. 'That is why I keep it in my private drawer.'

It was the first time that Mma Ramotswe had heard the term *private drawer* used to describe the drawers in Mma Makutsi's desk. And she could not see why her assistant should object so strongly to her looking in there, given that she had often found Mma Makutsi herself rifling through the drawers of her – Mma Ramotswe's – own desk, and had thought nothing of it. She knew that Mma Makutsi was not looking for anything personal, but was searching out a refill for a pen or a box of paper clips or something of that nature. That's what the drawers of office desks were for, was it not? And there was nothing personal about pen refills or boxes of paper clips. She was about to point this out to Mma Makutsi, but decided against it: there were times when an apology was best, she thought, even when one really had nothing to apologise for. If only people would say sorry sooner rather than later, Mma Ramotswe believed, much discord and unhappiness could be avoided. But that was not the way people were. So often pride stood in the way of apology, and then, when somebody was ready to say sorry, it was already too late.

'I'm very sorry, Mma Makutsi,' Mma Ramotswe said. 'I did not realise that that was your private drawer. I will not look for keys in there again.'

Mma Makutsi looked puzzled. 'What keys?' she asked. 'There are no keys in those drawers.'

'I needed to get into the filing cabinet,' explained Mma

Ramotswe. 'And you are the one who locks that. Maybe we should keep the key in some place where I can find it if I need it and you are not here.'

Mma Makutsi shook her head. 'I never lock the cabinet, Mma. I used to, but I don't any more. The key was bent and didn't fit very well, and so I do not lock the drawers.'

Mma Ramotswe moved over and gave the top drawer of the filing cabinet a tug. It did not budge. 'I think it is locked, Mma,' she said. 'Perhaps it has locked itself.'

And that was when Mma Ramotswe's earlier embarrassment over the photograph was compounded, as Mma Makutsi reached for the top drawer of the cabinet and gave it a sharp tug, at the same time pressing at the second drawer with her right knee.

'There, Mma, you see. You see – it opens.'

'So there is just a knack?'

'There is a just a knack.'

It was clear to Mma Ramotswe that even a cup of tea and a doughnut would not lift Mma Makutsi's mood, and so it was with some relief that she greeted Mr Polopetsi's popping his head round the door to inform her that he had finished his tasks in the garage and was free to accompany her on her mission. She explained to Mma Makutsi what she was going off to do, but Mma Makutsi still seemed sunk in her bad mood and so she eventually tiptoed out of the office as one would when somebody had a throbbing headache and found noise painful. It is my own office, she said to herself; and Mr Polopetsi, as he watched her leave, thought very much the same thing. She should tell that woman where the limits are, he thought; it is her own office and she is the one who pays her. I feel sorry for that poor man Phuti Radiphuti. Imagine being married to Mma Makutsi and having to look into those large glasses all the time. Poor man – it is the end for you, Phuti Radiphuti, it really is. The end.

Mma Sebina had been brought up in Otse, a village only twenty minutes or so out of Gaborone to the south. It was much smaller than Mochudi, the village where Mma Ramotswe had grown up, and even more intimate as a result. As Mma Ramotswe turned her van off the Lobatse Road, Mr Polopetsi asked how they would go about finding a friend of Mma Sebina's late mother.

Mma Ramotswe steered the van past a particularly large hole in the road. 'Well, Rra,' she said, 'I have always followed a very simple rule in these matters. When I want to find something out, I usually ask somebody directly. That is the best way to get information: you ask for it and it is given to you.'

Mr Polopetsi smiled. 'But do people always tell you the truth?'

Mma Ramotswe peered over the top of her steering wheel. 'Not always. But then you can tell when they're telling lies. If you watch people when they talk to you, you can tell.'

Mr Polopetsi turned to stare at her, and she met his gaze briefly before looking ahead again at the road. He had looked doubtful and it occurred to her that this was because of what had happened to him. His experience disproved what she said – he *knew* that people could not always tell the difference between lies and truth. He had been sent to prison because even a judge, who sits all day and listens to people giving conflicting versions of the truth, even such a person could not tell. Perhaps I claim too much, thought Mma Ramotswe; perhaps I cannot really tell.

They drove on and were soon passing through the outskirts of the village, past the small white-painted houses dotted here and there, past a herd-boy with a line of nibbling goats, past a sign pointing off to a butchery somewhere out in the bush. Then suddenly Mma Ramotswe applied the brakes and brought the tiny white van to a halt.

'You see that lady?' She pointed to a woman who was sitting in a chair under an acacia tree, just a few yards off the road. Above her, hanging from a branch overhead, but comfortably within reach, was another chair.

'There is a chair in the tree,' observed Mr Polopetsi. 'I wonder why . . .'

'I'm going to ask that lady,' said Mma Ramotswe. 'She is doing nothing, and she looks like a lady who knows things.'

They got out of the van and picked their way across the dusty strip of land that separated them from the woman under her acacia tree.

'*Dumela, Mma.*'

Greetings exchanged, Mma Ramotswe pointed up at the extra chair hanging on the branch above the woman's head. 'It is strange to see a chair in a tree, Mma.'

The woman looked up, as if seeing the chair for the first

time. 'Oh, that chair. That is a chair I keep for visitors, Mma. You see, I sell tomatoes here. I have a small stall, but there was a strong wind last week and it blew it away. I am sitting here because I have got so used to it.'

'You could make a new stall, Mma,' said Mr Polopetsi, gazing up at the chair.

'I will do that soon,' said the woman, 'but not just yet.' She looked down at her lap, where her hands were folded. 'My hands are not ready for work yet. They have been working, working, working. Now it is time for my hands to take a rest.'

Mma Ramotswe nodded her head in understanding. There was so much work for women in Africa: fields to be tilled, yards to be swept, clothes to be washed, children to be brought up. That was their lot, and they did it without complaint, without asking the men whether they would care to do some of this work that women did – not all of it, just some. And now here was this woman, her faded skirt cloth wrapped around her waist, taking a short break from all that work, sitting under her tree with the spare chair dangling above her head.

'I'm sure that your hands deserve a rest,' said Mma Ramotswe, glancing at Mr Polopetsi as she spoke. He was a hard-working man, of course, but he was the only representative of the world of men present under that tree and so he would have to shoulder some of the blame.

Mr Polopetsi shifted on his feet. 'Mma Ramotswe is right,' he said. 'Your hands surely deserve a rest, Mma. They can go to sleep now.'

At the mention of Mma Ramotswe's name, the woman

looked up sharply. 'Mma Ramotswe? You are Mma Ramotswe?'

Mma Ramotswe inclined her head briefly and emitted the sibilant *ee* of the Setswana yes. That yes could be made to sound anything from accepting to wildly enthusiastic. This time it sounded cautious, implying that she might well be Mma Ramotswe but people should not read too much into that.

'You are the lady detective?' asked the woman. 'The one who has that office behind the garage? That one?'

'That is who she is,' said Mr Polopetsi proudly.

The woman looked briefly at Mr Polopetsi and then looked away, as if discounting the reliability of any statement he might make. 'Is that true, Mma?'

'It is true,' said Mma Ramotswe. 'But I may not be the sort of detective you think I am. I am not a lady who deals with criminal business. That is the job of the Botswana police force. They do it very well. I have nothing to do with all that.'

The woman seemed disappointed. 'But you are still a detective?'

'Yes,' answered Mma Ramotswe. 'But I am a lady first and then I am a detective. So I just do the things which we ladies know how to do – I talk to people and find out what has happened. Then I try to solve the problems in people's lives. That is all I do.'

'But that is a big thing,' said the woman. 'There are many problems in our lives. Big ones sometimes.' She suddenly unfolded her resting hands and gestured in the air to illuminate the immensity of the problems which people faced.

Mma Ramotswe smiled. 'Small ones too, Mma. Sometimes big problems are really tiny ones when you look at them in the right way.' She glanced again at Mr Polopetsi. They would have to get back to the subject or she sensed that this woman would talk for rather a long time.

Mr Polopetsi came to the rescue. 'We are looking for somebody to tell us about a lady who lived in this village,' he said. 'She is late now, and her husband is late too. She was called Mma Sebina.'

The woman, who had been frowning in concentration as he spoke, now smiled broadly. She ignored Mr Polopetsi, though, addressing her reply to Mma Ramotswe. It was an odd habit, thought Mma Ramotswe, who had noticed. It was the same thing that the younger apprentice did; when answering a question from Mma Makutsi he would look at Mma Ramotswe or Mr J. L. B. Matekoni. It was a way of saying, *You don't really exist for me; not entirely.* 'But I knew her, Mma,' said the woman. 'I knew that lady well. I was her best friend for a long time. A long time.' Her gaze moved from Mma Ramotswe out to the bush beyond, so dry now at this time of the year; no grazing at all for the cattle and slim pickings even for the goats.

'Your best friend?'

'She was. I was very sad when she became late, Mma. When your friends die . . . you know how your heart feels. Like this.' She clenched her right fist tight: the human heart made small.

Mma Ramotswe was silent for a moment. She had not thought much about Mma Sebina's mother and what she was like; she had been interested only in finding out about how she had acquired the child all those years ago. But, of course, there would be a person at the end of that inquiry, a person who left others bereft on her passing. That was the trouble with any inquiry; one unravelled one piece of the skein and it revealed so many little strands, each of which was a story in itself.

She spoke gently. 'You must miss her, Mma,' she said. 'I know how it is to lose a close friend.'

The woman inclined her head in acknowledgement.

'And her daughter, Mma?' Mma Ramotswe continued. 'Tell me about her daughter.'

It took the woman some time to reply, and when she did her tone had changed from regret to something close to anger. 'That girl is no good. She was always complaining, complaining, complaining. Like one of those birds that goes on and on all day, telling us that some other bird has stolen its nest or the snake has eaten its eggs. That is what that girl is like.'

They were a bit taken aback. Mr Polopetsi lifted a hand to his mouth, as if he himself had suddenly spoken out of turn; Mma Ramotswe raised an eyebrow, but only just. 'I did not know that,' she said. 'Perhaps you could tell me about that, Mma.'

The woman drew in her breath. 'Oh, there is a lot to say, Mma. There is so much that I hardly know where to begin. She was an ungrateful girl – very ungrateful. That lady and her husband gave that girl everything. They paid big school fees – big like this – for her to go to school. They bought her pretty dresses and everything she wanted. When she was a little girl I remember her with her mouth full of sweeties all the time. Morning, afternoon. All the time.'

'And her teeth,' observed Mma Ramotswe, even as she thought, If I had been allowed to have my mouth full of sweeties all the time, how I would have loved it!

The woman looked blank. 'I do not see what that has to do with her teeth, Mma. I have not said anything about her teeth.'

Mr Polopetsi intervened. 'I think that Mma Ramotswe meant that if her mouth was always full of sweeties, then her teeth would have had many holes in them. Like those places where the rock rabbits live. Those places in the rocks where they make their holes.'

The woman stared at Mma Ramotswe. 'Why is he talking about rock rabbits now, Mma? Can you tell me?'

Mma Ramotswe exchanged a quick glance with Mr Polopetsi. He was well meaning, but he did not know that one should try to keep people on track when one was questioning them. Clovis Andersen himself made that point in his chapter on 'Getting to the Truth' in *The Principles of Private Detection*. 'Some people,' he wrote, 'cannot resist the opportunity to talk about things that have nothing to do with the case. They wander off in all sorts of directions and lose sight of the subject in hand. Don't fall into the trap of distracting them.'

'I don't think it matters much, Mma,' she said soothingly. 'I expect that he was thinking of something else. Now, why do you think this girl was ungrateful? If her parents were so kind to her, then why was she ungrateful?'

The woman reached out and laid a hand on Mma

Ramotswe's forearm. When she answered, she spoke in a low voice, so that Mr Polopetsi had to lean forward to hear what she said. This made the woman lower her voice even further. 'Her parents, you say, Mma. You say her parents. I say her parents. But that girl, she thought that they were not her parents at all! She said that herself. Not to everyone, but she said it to me once, and to another lady who knew her mother. And to a woman in the Women's Guild at the church. She said it. She said that she came from somewhere else.'

This revelation was greeted with complete silence. Then Mma Ramotswe spoke. 'And was this true, do you think?'

The woman suddenly stood up, straightening her skirt and brushing imagined dust off her sleeve. She looked up at the sky. 'It is going to rain, Mma. At long last it is going to rain.'

Mma Ramotswe glanced over her shoulder at the clouds that had built up to the east. They were heavy and purple, stacked in towering layers; so sudden, so welcome. 'Yes,' she said. 'That is very good. The land is very thirsty.' She reached out and touched the woman's shoulder. 'But tell me one thing, Mma, and then we will leave you to get on with your . . . with your resting. Tell me, was it true that this girl was the child of another lady?'

The woman laughed. 'Certainly not, Mma. It is certainly not true.'

'Can you be sure?' Mma Ramotswe probed.

Again the woman laughed. 'Can I be sure, Mma? Of course I can. I can be sure because I was there in the house when she gave birth. We had been friends since we were girls, and I helped her when she had her baby. It was myself and the woman from the village who helped at births. We were both there, and some other women too. All the women together. I saw that girl come out of her mother. I saw it myself.' She looked at Mma Ramotswe; there was something triumphant about her manner, the look of one who had laid a canard to rest. 'And I'll tell you something else, Mma. I saw the baby open her eyes for the first time – I was right there, as close as I am to you – and I saw the look in those eyes. It was a complaining look, and I said to myself, This one will do a lot of shouting. And, do you know, Mma, straight away that baby started to cry and make a fuss about being born. That is the sort of baby she was.'

They left the woman, but only after she had given them a list of other friends of the late Mma Sebina, senior. None of these women knew her as well as she did, of course, but she was sure that they would confirm what she had told them. And then, with the storm clouds now virtually upon them, they made their way back to the tiny white van.

'We can't go and look for these people in the rain,' said Mma Ramotswe, glancing up at the purple clouds. 'We shall have to come back.'

'We shall have to come back,' agreed Mr Polopetsi, who had a habit of repeating what was said to him; an innocuous enough habit, until one noticed it.

Mma Ramotswe turned the van and they had just started back when the first drops of rain began to fall. First there was that smell, that smell of rain, so unlike anything else, but immediately recognisable and enough to make the heart of a dry person soar; for that, thought Mma Ramotswe, is what we Batswana are: dry people, people who can live with dust and dryness but whose hearts dream of rain and water. Now, in great veils, the rain fell upon Botswana; great purple-white veils joining sky to land, soaking the parched landscape.

They drove down the road through the welcome deluge, travelling slowly for the puddles and sheets of water that were forming so quickly. The tiny white van, valiant in every sort of condition, ploughed through the water like an albino hippo, while its windscreen wipers swept backwards and forwards, making it possible, just, to see a few yards ahead through the downpour. But then, as if overcome by the sheer effort of pushing aside so much water, the wipers collided with one another and became stuck. Immediately Mma Ramotswe and Mr Polopetsi were as if shrouded in a completely impenetrable mist.

'I cannot carry on driving if I cannot see,' said Mma Ramotswe. 'We shall have to stop.'

She drew the van to the side of the road, or to what she hoped was the side of the road; it was impossible to see even that.

Mr Polopetsi rubbed at the steam on the passenger window with the sleeve of his jacket. 'I will get out and fix those, Mma,' he said. 'They are just stuck.'

Mma Ramotswe made a clucking sound with her tongue. 'You don't need to do that, Rra. You will get soaked. Wait until it eases a bit.'

Mr Polopetsi peered through the small circle he had cleared in the condensation. 'It will not clear quickly. This rain is going to go on for some time. I do not mind a bit of nice warm rain, Mma.' He turned to grin at her. 'Why should I mind that? We have waterproof skins, do we not, Mma? Is that not what God has given us?'

He reached for the door lever and flung the door open. She felt the rain come in as he got out of the van, and then he had slammed the door closed again. She saw him grappling with the windscreen wipers, which were recalcitrant. But eventually he freed them and they sprang back into operation again, describing their squeaky arcs in the still heavy rain.

When Mr Polopetsi clambered back into the van his outer clothing was soaked.

'Look at your jacket, Rra,' she said. 'You must take it off. Your shirt will be drier underneath.'

Mr Polopetsi was stoic. 'It's nothing,' he said. 'I shall get dry soon. Let's just go back now.'

Mma Ramotswe felt that she had to insist. She could see that his shirt was damp, but had not been soaked as thoroughly as his jacket. 'No,' she said, starting to tug at the neck and shoulders of the jacket. 'Come on now, take it off.'

He sighed. 'If you insist, Mma Ramotswe. If you insist.'

She smiled and continued to help him wriggle out of the jacket. 'It is for your own good, Rra. Women know about these things.'

The jacket was off his shoulders and she gave it a shake, constrained by the small cabin of the van, but enough to get some of the moisture out. As she did so, an envelope fell out of the pocket.

'A letter,' she said. 'I hope it is not wet.'

The letter had fallen on her lap, and she picked it up.

'Oh, it has my name on it,' she said. 'Look. Mma Ramotswe.'

Mr Polopetsi had become quite still. She heard his breathing, which sounded strange, as if he had just run up a flight of stairs. She looked down at the letter in her hands. It was definitely addressed to her. She slipped a finger under the flap and opened it.

Fat woman beware! You think that you are Number 1, but you are Number Nothing!

She read the letter in disbelief, in confusion. It was on the same paper as the last one; it was by the same hand. She looked up. Mr Polopetsi was staring at the letter.

'I found it in the garage. I picked it up and was going to give it to you.'

She looked again at the piece of paper. Outside, it seemed as if the rain had intensified; there was an insistent drumming on the roof of the van. Watery sounds. 'Found it?' she asked. 'Where?'

He seemed to hesitate for a moment. Then he said, 'I found it on one of the oil drums. You know that one by the side. Somebody must have left it there. It is a wicked letter, Mma. It is from some stupid person who doesn't know what he's writing.'

Mma Ramotswe folded the letter up carefully and tucked it

into her pocket. 'You said *he*, Rra. Why did you say *he*? Why do you think this letter is from a man?'

Again he hesitated before replying. 'Because the writers of such letters are usually men,' he said. 'It is the sort of letter that a stupid man writes.'

She looked ahead and engaged the van's gears slowly, tentatively, as if she was pondering something. 'You didn't know what was in it, did you, Rra?' she asked, looking at him as she spoke. The tiny white van strayed from its path, towards the middle of the road.

'Of course not, Mma,' said Mr Polopetsi. 'I would not read a letter addressed to *Mma Ramotswe*.'

Nor write one? she asked herself.

Chapter Seven

Look, the Heart is Bleeding

During Mma Ramotswe's absence with Mr Polopetsi, Mma Makutsi had spent her time tidying the office. It was a task that she always enjoyed, as she prided herself on being a ruthless disposer of unnecessary things. That was something that she had learned at the Botswana Secretarial College where it had been stressed time and time again – almost to the point of becoming a mantra – *A tidy office is an efficient office.* And they had been given examples of real-life cases where untidiness in an office had led to disaster. One of these was that of a firm of quantity surveyors who had lost the contract for the construction of a large dam when the carefully prepared tender documents had gone missing in their notoriously untidy office. There had not been time to prepare another set before the deadline and the contract had gone to a rival. 'Later on,' said the lecturer, 'the documents were found under the chair of the head secretary. She had been sitting on them.'

That had brought laughter, even from Violet Sephotho, the undisputed ringleader of the glamorous girls in Mma Makutsi's year; she, who normally heard very little of what was going on, so busy was she with the painting of her nails in the back row. She it was who had walked into a well-paid job with her miserable fifty-one per cent or whatever it was, while Mma Makutsi, with her distinguished record, had been turned down, sometimes with not so much as an interview.

No, Mma Makutsi was not one to clutter, and she had soon built up a small pile of things that she judged ready to go. There was a box of old pencils that Mma Ramotswe had salvaged, but never used; that would not be missed. There were several promotional writing pads, given to Mr J. L. B. Matekoni by a tyre salesman, that had been ignored on a shelf and were now yellowed with age. There were various items of evidence garnered in old investigations: a tie left behind in a room and then discovered by a suspicious husband; the tie of a paramour, a thin, brightly coloured tie, that *looked* guilty. 'A man who would wear a tie like that could do *anything*,' Mma Ramotswe had observed.

Mma Makutsi gathered the items together and began to look around for something to put them in. Then she saw the rain clouds, and moved over to the window to look out at them. It was the sight that everybody was waiting for; the beginnings of a rainy season, they hoped, that would bring life to the land again. Rain was what mattered in Botswana – mattered above all else.

Mma Makutsi sent up a silent prayer. This season had to be good, or the level in the great dam that held Gaborone's water would remain perilously low. And if that happened, there would be water rationing again and people's gardens, such as they were, would wither and give up. But her prayer was not for Gaborone, but for the north, for her people up in Bobonong, who needed the rain more desperately than she did. For them, good rains meant fat cattle and sleek goats, not to mention good yields of sorghum for the making of flour.

And then it started. There was a wind and a movement in the trees, followed by the rain. Mma Makutsi saw the first drops hit the white earth of the garage yard, throwing up what looked like tiny worms of water and sand. Then these merged into one and became a silver shimmer of rapidly growing puddles; even the thirsty earth could not absorb this sudden munificence of water. She saw Mr J. L. B. Matekoni running through the rain to his truck, sheltering his head with an old newspaper. He had urgent business to attend to, it seemed; a car stuck in the rain somewhere? A window left open at home and suddenly remembered—

The appalling thought struck her – the new bed – and she screamed. She had left her handsome new bed in the open, stacked against the side wall of the house, and now . . . She gave another cry and ran to the door. The two apprentices were standing near the front of the garage, watching the downpour. One of them, Charlie, was whittling away at a small stick with his penknife when Mma Makutsi called out as she ran towards him.

'Charlie! You have to drive me. I need to go home. Now. Right now.'

Charlie looked up from his whittling. 'Why not wait? This will not last very long.' He made some additional remark to the younger apprentice, which Mma Makutsi did not hear properly but which sounded like, 'I am not a taxi service.'

She bit her tongue. No, indeed, he was not a taxi service. He had been one, though, and had crashed the taxi on the first day, but she felt that it would not be helpful to mention that now.

'Please, Charlie,' she begged. 'I have left something out in the rain. I have left a bed outside.'

Charlie smiled. 'Then it will have become a water bed, Mma,' he said. 'They are very fashionable and expensive. You have made one for nothing now.' He glanced at the younger apprentice for an appreciation of his wit. There was a smile of encouragement.

Mma Makutsi resisted the strong temptation to reach out and slap this annoying young man. 'Charlie,' she said, 'if you do not take me, I shall walk out in this storm and I will be struck by lightning. But before I walk out, I shall hide a note in the office saying, *If I become late – for any reason, even if it's made to look like an act of God – it is Charlie's fault.*'

The look of confidence on Charlie's face faded. 'They will know it was lightning—'

Mma Makutsi cut him off. 'I can see that you are not a detective,' she said. 'I can see that. How do you know that lightning has struck if nobody saw what happened? Lightning comes and goes – bang, like that.'

'You would be burned up,' said Charlie. 'There would be big electricity marks.'

'Big electricity marks?' Mma Makutsi mocked. 'And what are those, can you tell me?'

'Burns,' said Charlie.

Mma Makutsi was silent for a moment. Then she smiled the smile of one who knew something that another did not. 'That's what you think,' she said. 'Well, it's obvious that you have never dealt with a case of lightning. That is very obvious.' She said no more; she had not dealt with a case of lightning either, but how was Charlie to know that?

The younger apprentice looked nervous. 'You should take Mma Makutsi, Charlie,' he urged. 'I do not want her to be struck by lightning.'

'Thank you,' said Mma Makutsi. 'I would not like that to happen to *you* either.' The *you* was pointed, and plainly excluded Charlie; it was clear that her concern as to the control of lightning damage was limited, and that beyond that the forces of nature could do their worst.

Charlie hesitated, and then reluctantly agreed. 'We must go now, though, Mma,' he said. 'We cannot stand about here discussing it.'

Again Mma Makutsi had to struggle to control herself. She had not asked for any discussion and it was Charlie who had caused the delay. She closed her eyes and swallowed hard. 'Thank you, Charlie,' she said. 'You are very kind.' It was what Mma Ramotswe would probably have said, and she wondered, for a moment, if she was suddenly acquiring Mma Ramotswe's patience. But no, she decided, she would never be as understanding as her employer, especially when it came to Charlie, who would try the patience of a saint, even if not that of Mma Ramotswe.

They ran out, ignoring the rain, and set off in Mr J. L. B. Matekoni's towing truck. 'I'm sorry about your bed,' Charlie said. 'I would not like you to think that I was not sorry for you, Mma.'

Mma Makutsi inclined her head. 'Thank you. I feel very silly about it. I did not think it would rain today. I was not thinking.'

'Nobody knew that there would be rain,' said Charlie. 'Everybody thought that it would go on being dry.'

'And we should never complain about rain,' said Mma Makutsi. 'It would be a very dangerous thing for a Motswana to complain about rain.'

Charlie agreed; that would be unheard of. 'This is very good rain,' he said, negotiating a small lake of floodwater that had built up beside the road.

Mma Makutsi said nothing. She was thinking of what she would find at the end of the journey, which she was sure would be a sodden mess. Oh, if only she had thought! Who would leave a bed, of all things, outside, exposed to the elements? Well, the answer to that was she would, as she had just done.

She directed Charlie down the narrow road that led to her house. Any hopes she might have cherished that the rain in this part of town might have been gentler were dashed by the sight of the large puddles of mud-brown water beside the road and, on occasion, on it. Although the rain itself was now easing off, there was no doubt that there had been as much of a downpour here as anywhere else; perhaps more.

'That is my house,' she said in a subdued tone, pointing it out to Charlie.

'It is a nice place, Mma,' said Charlie. 'I wouldn't mind living in a place like that. At the moment I'm staying . . .' He tailed off. They had both seen the bed at the same time, and were now staring at the drooping, sodden item propped up against the side of the house.

Mma Makutsi groaned. 'It is ruined,' she said. 'It is completely ruined.'

There was no sign of Charlie's jaunty cheekiness as they alighted from the truck and walked up the small path that led to Mma Makutsi's house.

'I'm so sorry, Mma,' said Charlie. 'I don't think the rain has done the bed any good. Was it an old one?'

Mma Makutsi stared at the bed that had been her pride and joy. 'It was brand new,' she said, her voice faltering with emotion. 'It had never been slept in. Not once.'

Charlie poked at the surface of the velvet heart-shaped

headboard. He did not exert much pressure, but the water-logged cloth gave way under his finger, exposing sodden padding-material behind. He picked at this, twisted it between his fingers, and then dropped it. 'What is this red bit, Mma? Or should I say, what *was* it?'

'A heart,' muttered Mma Makutsi. 'The headboard was a heart.'

'Why?' asked Charlie. 'Why have a heart?'

Mma Makutsi did not answer. She had moved round to examine the side of the bed. The rain, she saw, had penetrated everywhere and there was a steady dripping of water from the lower edge of the mattress. She hardly dared raise her eyes to the velvet heart, but she did so now and saw that the water dripping from that part of the ruined bed was dyed red, as if it were blood. And she said to Charlie, in her sorrow, 'Look, the heart is bleeding,' and he reached out and touched her lightly on the shoulder. It was an uncharacteristically sympathetic gesture from the young man, who was normally all jokes and showing-off, but who now, in the face of this little tragedy, proved himself capable of understanding, and did.

Chapter Eight

As if the World itself was Broken

When Mma Ramotswe arrived back at the office, having dropped Mr Polopetsi off at his home, there was no sign of Mma Makutsi. The office door was unlocked, and the younger apprentice said that Mma Makutsi and Charlie had dashed off together to deal with something that had been left out in the rain. They had not said when they would be back.

'And Mr J. L. B. Matekoni?' asked Mma Ramotswe. 'Has he been washed away too?'

The apprentice thought this very funny. 'He went off in his truck. He said that there was a car, an important car, that would not start because of the rain and he had gone to fix it.

There are some cars that do not like all this rain, Mma. You see, the water can get in the distributor – you know what a distributor is, do you, Mma? It is the part that sends the electricity to the—'

'Yes, yes,' said Mma Ramotswe. 'Women know about distributors these days. But why has everybody gone off like this? What if a client were to come here?'

The apprentice shook his head. 'There have been no clients, Mma. I have not seen any and I have been here all the time except when I went off to the shops for some meat.'

Mma Ramotswe sighed. She had spoken to people about the importance of not leaving the business unattended, but nobody, it seemed, listened. Mr J. L. B. Matekoni heard what she had to say, perhaps, but was such a kind man that he would often disappear at the drop of a hat if one of the customers of Tlokweng Road Speedy Motors was in any sort of trouble. Mma Potokwani, of course, knew this full well, and would not hesitate to impose upon him to fix anything that went wrong at the orphan farm, but there were others as well, presumably including this person who had summoned him in the middle of the thunderstorm purely because his car would not start.

She sighed again. It was no use thinking about it and getting hot under the collar because whatever she said she would never be able to change the way people were. Of course she believed in the *possibility* of change; she had seen many who had become better people from a single experience or from the example of another, but that change was in the big matters, change in the outlook of the heart. It was not change in the little things of life, such as leaving the business unattended – those were things which never changed.

The rain had now eased off and the sky in the east, which had been dark purple with the storm, was now light again, although there was still cloud, great banks of it, white now, touched gold by the sun, and a rainbow, too, arched over the land and dipping down like a pointer to the horizon somewhere beyond Mochudi.

The apprentice, standing beside her, suddenly tugged excitedly at the sleeve of her dress. 'Look, Mma Ramotswe! Look!'

She looked in the direction in which he was pointing and immediately saw what he had seen. Flying ants. Suddenly, unexpectedly, the air was filling with flying ants, rising up from their secret burrows in the rain-softened ground, gaining altitude on beating wings, dipping down again. It was a familiar sight following the rains, one of those sights that took one back to childhood no matter what age one was, and brought to mind memories of chasing these ants, grabbing them from the air, and then eating them, for their peanut-butter taste and crunchiness.

'Go and catch some,' she said to the apprentice.

He handed her the spanner he was holding and rushed out in the last few drops of rain to snatch at the termites, a boy again. He caught some easily, and de-winged them before stuffing them into his mouth. Above him there were other, hungrier dangers for the ants; a flock of swifts, materialising from nowhere, had swept in and were dipping and swooping over their aerial feast. The apprentice looked up at the birds and watched them, and smiled; and she smiled back. What does it matter, she thought, if businesses are left unattended, if people are not always as we want them to be; we need the time just to be human, to enjoy something like this: a boy chasing ants, a dry land drinking at last, birds in the sky, a rainbow.

She stayed at the office for half an hour or so, enough time to brew herself a pot of red bush tea and to set her thoughts in order. The accidental discovery of the letter in the van had shocked and disturbed her. Mr Polopetsi's explanation of having found the letter in the garage was feasible enough but there had been something about the manner in which he had made these protestations that did not ring true. He had hesitated, and when people hesitated it meant that either they were lying, or they were thinking about your reaction to what they were about to say. But if she gave Mr Polopetsi the benefit of the doubt and decided that he was hesitant merely because he feared her reaction to his explanation, she still had to answer why he would have harboured this fear. There was nothing wrong in what he had done – picking up a letter addressed to her and pocketing it with a view to passing it on later; so why should he have been furtive? It did not make sense, and that meant that he must have written the letter himself. It was an appalling conclusion – one that made her sit quite still, her head in her hands, even letting her cup of bush tea get cold, as she pondered the enormity of what she had inadvertently discovered: she had an enemy in the heart of the No. 1 Ladies' Detective Agency, somebody whom she had trusted. And what had she done to deserve that? She could not answer that question. Pick as she might over all her dealings with the seemingly innocuous Mr Polopetsi, she could not think of a single thing that she had done which would justify his enmity; not one thing. But then she thought: enmity does not require an unjust act to bring it into existence; sometimes simple envy is quite enough. Envy extended its tentacles into the chambers of the human heart, strangled what it found. Mr Polopetsi was a poor man who had suffered great injustice – now he had so very little, while she had so much. That was what must have turned him. There might be an explanation for his behaviour, then, but that was very different from there being an excuse.

Mma Ramotswe shivered. The rain had lowered the temperature and the office was cool and dark. The sky had darkened again, grey shading into cloud-white; the sun had disappeared. She was alone in the office now, with only the apprentice outside, and, in the distance, the sound of cars moving through flooded sections of the road, some with their headlights still on from the storm. The absence of sun disconcerted her; it was as if the country was suddenly out of favour, deserted by its constant daytime companion.

She tried to work, making a list of the names she had been given by the woman in Otse – the names of Mma Sebina senior's friends in Gaborone. The act of writing these down brought home to her that the investigation was posing a fundamental dilemma: whether or not to believe the client. This was one of the most difficult situations that somebody in her position could face. If the client was lying – for whatever reason – then the whole premise upon which inquiries were based could be false. And in this case it looked as if any time spent on meeting and talking to the friends of Mma Sebina's mother would be wasted. There would be more point, she thought, in trying to persuade Mma Sebina to come to terms with the fact that her mother really was her mother. That is what Mma Ramotswe felt she should do, although she wondered *why* she should do it. Of course the answer to that was that Mma Ramotswe was there to help people, and anybody who was actively denying that her mother was her mother surely needed some help.

She set aside the list and looked up at the ceiling. The place where rainwater had previously penetrated the roof was now damp again. It was not something to worry about unduly; rain was so infrequent in Botswana that a leaky roof simply was not a problem. And if the water stained the ceiling board, then it would merely add to the many other marks up there – the places where insects had died, the sites of struggles between flies and geckos, the tiny battle grounds. A dripping of water was a flood of biblical proportions for the creatures of the ceiling, but nothing of any importance to the people below.

Mma Ramotswe's musings were interrupted by the sound of Mr J. L. B. Matekoni's truck returning. She could always tell when he came back, as the truck's engine had a particular note to it – a whining sound that he insisted was quite normal but seemed to her to be an indication of mechanical trouble of some sort. And Charlie thought so too, as he had raised it with Mr J. L. B. Matekoni at tea one morning and had been told that there was nothing wrong.

'I think you are in denial, Boss,' Charlie had said.

Mr J. L. B. Matekoni looked puzzled. 'Denial? What am I denying? You're the one who's in denial, Charlie. What about those exams you have to take if you are to finish your apprenticeship? What about those?'

'I will do those exams some day, Boss. They will still be there.'

Mr J. L. B. Matekoni said, 'Then you will never finish your apprenticeship. You will be the oldest apprentice in the country. In fact, you will be a retired apprentice eventually.'

Charlie ignored this. 'There is something wrong with your truck, Rra. I can hear it. Even Mma Ramotswe can hear it, and she is just a woman.'

Mma Ramotswe had let that pass; there was no point in engaging with Charlie on these matters, she thought. And Charlie was right about the truck and its engine sound. There was something wrong, even if Mr J. L. B. Matekoni seemed unwilling to face it.

The engine was switched off and the whining stopped. A few moments later Mr J. L. B. Matekoni put his head round the door. 'Wonderful rain, Mma Ramotswe. You should see the storm drains up near Maru-a-Pula – they were like a big river. Like the Limpopo itself. That much water.'

She nodded. 'It is very good. Maybe we'll have a good season this year.'

'We can hope.'

She looked at her husband, noticing that his shirt was wet and was sticking to his skin. There was something strange about his manner; something almost elated. Was he just pleased about the rain, she wondered, or was there something else? 'You must dry yourself off, Rra,' she said. 'You shouldn't stand around in wet clothes.'

'Rain harms nobody,' said Mr J. L. B. Matekoni. 'And I am not that wet. Just a little.'

There was still something about him, something she could not put her finger on. The apprentice had told her that he had rushed off to start an important car and now he was back, looking as if something nice had happened to him.

'Where have you been, Mr J. L. B. Matekoni? You are looking very happy, I think.'

He smiled. 'I have been to help somebody with his car. It would not start and he had to get somewhere in a hurry. I managed to get it started.'

She waited for further explanation, but none came.

'Whose car?'

He frowned. Mr J. L. B. Matekoni did not like to be quizzed: 'I am not one of your suspects,' he had protested once. 'You must not talk to me with your detective shoes on.'

'One of my customers,' he said.

'I see.' She fixed him with her gaze, and he shifted on his feet.

'He is a doctor.'

She did not lower her gaze. 'Dr Moffat? You've been helping Dr Moffat?'

'No,' he said. 'Not him. Another doctor.' He paused, and then suddenly moved across the room, picked up the client's chair, moved it to the front of Mma Ramotswe's desk, and sat down.

'There is something we need to talk about,' he said, leaning forward in the chair. 'It is very important.'

Mma Ramotswe felt her heart miss a beat. Something very important. He was ill; that was it. And yet there was this look about him, this look of excitement. If he was ill, then surely he would look despondent.

She remembered suddenly what Dr Moffat had told her when he had treated Mr J. L. B. Matekoni for depression a few years earlier. 'Sometimes this illness comes with periods of elation,' he had said. 'A person can feel very excited, very cheerful. He can rush round on all sorts of wild schemes, thinking he can conquer the world. You have to watch for that.'

She had never seen that in Mr J. L. B. Matekoni, but now she found herself wondering whether this was what was happening. She tried to keep her voice steady as she told him that she was ready to listen; he could tell her whatever it was that he needed to tell her.

He looked her in the eyes. 'I went to see this doctor,' he said.

He could take a long time to tell a story. Often there was a lot of background information before he got started. She would be patient. 'Yes. The one with the car that wouldn't start? You went to see him.'

'He is a good man,' he went on. 'He was a doctor up in Selebi-Phikwe, at the mines, but now he is retired. He is living just outside town. Near David Mgang's place. Out that way.'

There were some big houses out there, thought Mma Ramotswe. This doctor had done well for himself. But she did not say that; she just said, 'Out there. I know that place.'

'Yes,' said Mr J. L. B. Matekoni. 'He has a nice place out there. His wife is late, but he has a son and his son's wife living with him, and there are many grandchildren. All in that house.'

'They must be happy,' said Mma Ramotswe. 'It is a good thing to have one's grandchildren around you when you have finished working. You can see the results of all your hard work then.'

He nodded, and then became silent. It was as if he was thinking about the grandchildren, and the rewards of hard work.

'So?' said Mma Ramotswe gently.

The verbal nudge seemed to focus him again. 'Yes,' he said. 'After I had got the car going, the doctor asked me whether I had a wife.'

Mma Ramotswe nodded encouragingly. 'And you said?'

'I said, yes, I have a wife.'

'I am relieved,' she said.

'And then he asked me whether I had any children. And I said there were no children of our own, but that we had the two foster-children, and they were like a son and a daughter. I told him that Motholeli was in a wheelchair but that she was doing well. And then . . .'

She was watching him. Now his eyes seemed to light up with pleasure.

'And then?'

Mr J. L. B. Matekoni leaned forward again. She noticed that the moisture from the rain had penetrated the cap of the pen which he had been carrying in his pocket so that the ink had run into the fabric of his shirt. That would be a difficult stain to remove; she would have to soak the shirt.

'And then he asked me what was wrong with her and I told him. I told him what they had said at the hospital, that there had been . . .'

He stumbled on the term, as if to utter it brought pain. *Transverse myelitis of the spinal cord, leading to paralysis.* She had looked at those words on the doctor's letter so many times; she knew them so well. They were the words in which the sentence had been delivered; the sentence that meant that Motholeli would be in her wheelchair for the rest of her life.

Mr J. L. B. Matekoni repeated the name of the condition slowly, forcing his tongue round the awkward syllables. Then he sat back. 'And he said that he had seen cases of that before.'

Mma Ramotswe was non-committal. 'I see. He knew about it.'

Mr J. L. B. Matekoni nodded his head eagerly. 'Then he said something very strange, Mma – something very exciting. He said, "I have dealt with cases like that. I have dealt with them satisfactorily." Those were his exact words. That is what he said.'

She did not move. 'Satisfactorily?'

'Yes, satisfactorily. That very word.' He paused, watching the effect of what he was saying. Mma Ramotswe was quite still. 'Then he said – remember he is a doctor, Mma – then he said, "You bring that child to me and I can get her to walk again." That is what he said, Mma Ramotswe. That is what he said. I am not making it up, I promise you. *I can get her to walk again*. I am telling the truth.'

Of course you are telling the truth, thought Mma Ramotswe. And then she muttered, Oh, and then, Oh, again, and closed her eyes. She wanted Motholeli to walk again – she would have given anything for that. But they had been told in the clearest terms by the doctors at the Princess Marina Hospital that this would never happen precisely because it *could* not happen. Dr Moffat had explained it to them, too, when she had raised it while having tea with his wife. He always spoke quietly, so quietly that people had to strain to catch what he was saying, but she had heard every word of what he had said on that occasion. 'Once the infection has done its damage to the spinal cord, there is nothing that can be done. It is like a rope that has been cut in two. I'm sorry.'

And she had said, 'But can you not tie a rope together again?' She had said, 'A rope can be mended.'

'Then it is not like a rope,' he said. 'It is different.'

Mrs Moffat had taken her hand, for comfort, and they had sat there in silence for a while. Sometimes it seemed as if the world itself was broken, that there was something wrong with all of us, something broken in such a way that it might not be put together again; but the holding of hands, human hand in human hand, could help, could make the world seem less broken.

Chapter Nine

Mma Ramotswe Goes to Mochudi, that Place She Knows so Well

The next morning, when Mma Makutsi and Mma Ramotswe looked at one another across their desks, each felt herself to be the bearer of a heavy burden: each woman wanted to talk to the other, to seek advice and reassurance, but neither wanted to raise the subject of her distress. Mma Ramotswe thought of Mma Makutsi, 'She has not slept well, and now she is tired; something is preying on her mind; she can never hide it.' And Mma Makutsi thought of Mma Ramotswe, 'Something is worrying her, too. I can always tell. When Mma Ramotswe is worried, it is written on her face, in very big letters.'

For a few minutes they both pretended that all was well. Mma Makutsi, who had collected the mail from the post box, slit open the letters before putting them on her employer's desk. 'There is nothing interesting,' she said. 'These are all bills, I think, Mma. That one is the water bill. And that one is the telephone bill. It is a day of bills. It is not a day of cheques.'

Mma Ramotswe gazed at the envelopes. She always paid her bills promptly, but this morning she simply left them where they were, to be attended to later. Mma Makutsi, watching her, decided to speak. 'I hope you don't mind my saying it, Mma, but you are sad. There is something that is making your heart very heavy.'

Mma Ramotswe looked up. 'And you, too, Mma. We are both sad today.'

For a moment or two nothing further was said. Then Mma Ramotswe rose from her desk and shut the door into the garage. She turned and faced her assistant, who was looking at her expectantly.

'There is nobody out there to hear us, Mma Ramotswe,' Mma Makutsi said. 'There is just Charlie and the other one – and Mr Polopetsi, of course. Nobody else.'

Mma Ramotswe made a silencing gesture, raising a finger to her lips. How easily could Mr Polopetsi be misread. 'Mr Polopetsi,' she whispered. 'Mr Polopetsi.'

Mma Makutsi glanced at the door, as if she half expected Mr Polopetsi to be listening on the other side, his ear stuck to the keyhole.

'Mr Polopetsi?'

Mma Ramotswe nodded. 'Those letters,' she said, her voice still lowered. 'Those threatening letters.' She paused. She had not intended to voice her suspicions to Mma Makutsi but now she felt that she had to. 'He wrote them. It was Mr Polopetsi.'

Mma Makutsi let out a cry of surprise. Immediately she put a hand to her mouth in a gesture that was halfway between incredulity and shock.

'Yes,' Mma Ramotswe continued, glancing over her shoulder in the direction of the garage. 'When we were in the van I took his coat for him and another letter dropped out of his pocket. He said that he had picked it up and was going to give it to me, but he was very evasive. I could tell that what he said was not true.'

Mma Makutsi's eyes showed her disbelief. 'Surely not. Surely not him.'

Mma Ramotswe would have liked to agree. Surely it could not be the mild, inoffensive Mr Polopetsi, but how could she ignore the evidence of her own eyes? 'Well, the letter was in his pocket.'

Mma Makutsi shook her head. It was impossible, she argued. Mr Polopetsi was simply not a man to write a threatening letter to anybody. 'It would be like . . . be like being threatened by a . . . by a rabbit, Mma. Yes, by a rabbit. Rabbits do not write threatening letters.'

Mma Ramotswe had to smile at Mma Makutsi's turn of phrase. Her assistant sometimes said extraordinary things, but every now and then she made some remark that described a situation beautifully. This was such a one. Mr Polopetsi a rabbit . . . of course he was. But even if a rabbit were to write a threatening letter, might one not be frightened? After all, how was one to know that the letter came from a rabbit?

'I don't know, Mma,' said Mma Ramotswe. 'I think that it was him, but I can't think why he should have done it. Why? What have we done to harm Mr Polopetsi?'

Mma Makutsi shrugged, her initial surprise fading into indifference. She herself had not been frightened by that ridiculous letter and if this was the problem that was worrying Mma Ramotswe, then Mma Ramotswe's trouble was a minor one when compared with her own. 'Ask him,' she said. 'Just ask him whether he wrote them. See what he says.'

Of course Mma Ramotswe had thought of this, but she felt that she could not challenge Mr Polopetsi directly, no matter how damning the evidence against him seemed. She explained this to Mma Makutsi, reminding her that Mr Polopetsi had already been wrongly accused once in his life – and had suffered imprisonment for it – so that she could not take the risk of making a second, possibly false, accusation. It was likely, she thought, that he was the writer of the letters, but it was still far from certain, and there was a difference between the likely and the certain. 'How would he feel, Mma? How would he feel if he was telling the truth and I came up to him and accused him? How would he feel?'

'But what if he thinks that you suspect him but aren't saying anything? Won't that be every bit as bad, Mma Ramotswe?'

'I don't believe he thinks that.'

Mma Makutsi was not convinced. 'If you like, Mma,' she

said, 'I can ask him for you. It won't be so hard for him if he thinks that I am the one who suspects him. I am not his boss – I am just an associate detective.' She hesitated and Mma Ramotswe thought for a moment that she was going to raise the subject of promotion. It was bound to come up sooner or later and could easily occur in the midst of a discussion of something quite unconnected, such as the guilt, or innocence perhaps, of Mr Polopetsi.

'No,' said Mma Ramotswe hurriedly. 'I don't think so, Mma.' She had been standing beside Mma Makutsi's desk during this conversation, and now she went back to her own chair and sat down. Now that she had confessed what was troubling her, she felt concern for Mma Makutsi. Sometimes her assistant was moody for no particular reason, but she did not think that this was one of those occasions. 'And you, Mma Makutsi,' she said. 'What about you? There is something troubling you, isn't there?'

Mma Ramotswe listened in silence to the tale of woe that came tumbling out. Mma Makutsi described the purchase of the bed – 'such an unusual bed, Mma, with its heart-shaped headboard and its double-thickness mattress'. She listened as Mma Makutsi told her of the failed attempt to get the bed through the door and the realisation that it would have to be taken elsewhere, perhaps to Phuti's house, which was altogether larger and more accommodating.

'If only I had phoned him and told him,' she said, her voice heavy with misery. 'If only I had done that, Mma. He would have sent one of his trucks to pick it up and store it safely. But no, I didn't do that. I just left it there, Mma, although I knew as well as anybody that it was the beginning of the rainy season. Oh, I am a very stupid woman, Mma.'

Mma Ramotswe raised a hand. 'Stop, Mma Makutsi. You cannot say that. You are *not* a stupid woman. Would a stupid woman have got ninety-seven per cent? Would she?'

Mma Makutsi looked doubtful. Mma Ramotswe was right about ninety-seven per cent: it was not the mark of a stupid woman. 'Well, I was thoughtless on that occasion – put it that way, Mma. I just didn't think.'

'Anybody can forget something, Mma,' said Mma Ramotswe. 'We are human, after all.'

That, thought Mma Makutsi, was true. We were all human, even Mma Ramotswe herself, who was so kind and understanding and so quick with her forgiveness; even Mma Ramotswe could forget things and make mistakes. Her marriage to Note Mokoti had been a mistake, a big mistake, and there was that time she hit the tree when she was trying to park her tiny white van, and the occasion when she had put the wrong piece of paper in an envelope and sent a letter intended for person A to person B. That had been an unfortunate mistake, as in the letter to person A she had said that she thought it was person B who was stealing from the petty cash in person A's office; very unfortunate, but very effective, as person B, alarmed at the discovery of his misdeeds, had immediately run away. That had sorted out the problem, but it was a mistake none the less.

Remembering the mistakes, Mma Makutsi smiled.

'Why are you smiling?' asked Mma Ramotswe. 'Do you not agree with what I said about mistakes?'

'Oh, I do agree,' said Mma Makutsi. 'I agree with you, Mma. It's just that I was thinking about ...' She hesitated for a moment before continuing, 'I was thinking about your mistakes.'

Mma Ramotswe was not offended. 'I have made many of those,' she said. 'I have made some very bad mistakes. I cannot hide that fact.'

'Do you remember that letter?' asked Mma Makutsi. 'The one in which you said—'

Mma Ramotswe sank her head in her hands. 'Oh no, Mma! Please do not remind me of that. I feel all hot and bothered when anybody reminds me of that.'

'But it had a good result anyway,' said Mma Makutsi.

Mma Ramotswe nodded. 'Yes, sometimes mistakes can be a good thing. You might be in town and you mean to go into one shop and you go into another. And then you find a very old friend in that other shop. Or you meet the person you're going to marry – something like that.'

Mma Makutsi thought about this. There were so many decisions we made that at the time seemed very minor matters, but that could change the whole shape of our lives. 'Yes, Mma, you are right. In my case, if I had not forgotten my pencil box at school and gone back for it one afternoon, we would not be sitting here today. That little decision to go back and fetch it changed my life.'

Mma Ramotswe was interested. The gloom that had

descended on the office seemed to have lifted now and it seemed that they were getting back to normal; this meandering conversation had restored their spirits, and a cup of red bush tea would do the rest. 'Tell me about it, Mma. Tell me what happened, while you are putting on the kettle.'

Mma Makutsi rose from her desk and filled the kettle at the sink in the corner of the room. It was a story that she had told others countless times, but had not related to Mma Ramotswe. 'I had left my pencil box behind and could not do my homework. I was sixteen then and I was just about to sit my Cambridge, so it was very important that I did lots of work. So I turned round and began to walk back towards the school. It was a hot day, Mma, I remember that. It was really hot.

'It took me about half an hour. When I reached the school, it was quiet. You know how schools are when everybody has gone home. There is a smell of chalk and just that silence, silence, nothing.'

Mma Ramotswe nodded. *Silence, silence, nothing.* Yes, that was it.

'I was worried that the classroom doors would be locked, but they were not. In those days we didn't worry about locking, did we, Mma? Nobody locked anything in Botswana. The whole country had no locks on it.'

Again Mma Ramotswe nodded. *The whole country had no locks on it.* Mma Makutsi was right; she often expressed herself in an unusual way, but she was right. *The whole country had no locks on it;* yes, that was true, and we loved one another then. We still do, of course, Mma Ramotswe thought, but it is different. Perhaps there was not so much love as there was in those days. Perhaps our love was running out.

Mma Makutsi stood beside the kettle, watching it. *A watched kettle* . . . thought Mma Ramotswe, but did not give voice to the proverb. Mma Makutsi liked to question proverbs and would point out that of course watched kettles did boil – eventually.

They were back in Bobonong. 'I went into the classroom,' Mma Makutsi continued, 'and I found my pencil box. Then, as I was leaving, one of the teachers came in. She was surprised to see me, and at first I think that she thought I was stealing something. But when I told her that I had just come in to fetch my pencil box she understood. She was a nice teacher, that one; I had always liked her.

'She had an envelope in her hand and she took a leaflet out of it. "I have just received this," she said. "It is from the Botswana Secretarial College. They are writing to us about a scholarship they have set up – for half the fees. The principal is from up here, from Bobonong, and she wants a bright girl from this school to apply, somebody whose work is very neat."

'It took me a few moments to realise that she was suggesting me. Nobody had ever thought before that I could win something, and now this teacher was saying that I could be the girl who got that scholarship. My heart was like this, Mma, big like this. I was very happy.'

Mma Ramotswe was touched by this story. 'You must have been very happy, Mma. And you won that scholarship?'

Mma Makutsi nodded. 'Yes, I won it. And my family paid

the other half of the fees. They sold some animals to do it. They sold some goats.'

Mma Ramotswe knew what that meant. The sale of cattle, of goats, inevitably took a family closer to the edge of survival; it was a serious matter. 'They must have been very proud of you, Mma. And they must be proud, too, now that you are engaged to a man like Phuti Radiphuti . . .'

She had meant to be reassuring, but it was the wrong thing to say; one had to be so careful with Mma Makutsi, who could so readily take things the wrong way. The younger woman's face crumpled. 'But what are we going to do, Mma Ramotswe?' she wailed. 'Phuti is coming back from Serowe in a couple of days. He has been up there on business. What am I to do when he comes back? I cannot face him and tell him that I have destroyed our expensive new bed. I cannot face him, Mma Ramotswe. What will he think of me?'

Mma Ramotswe thought for a moment. Phuti seemed to her to be an understanding man; surely he would not be vindictive about the loss of a bed. But then men were unpredictable; even outwardly mild men could suddenly become unreasonable. She pointed to the teapot. 'First things first, Mma,' she said. 'Tea helps us to think things through.'

They sat with their cups of tea. Mma Ramotswe took a sip of red bush, and Mma Makutsi raised her cup of ordinary tea to her mouth, anxiously, unenthusiastically.

'I could tell him,' said Mma Ramotswe. 'I could do it. If you are too embarrassed, then let me tell him. That is the simplest solution.'

'Oh, Mma,' said Mma Makutsi. 'If you would do that . . . I know that I am being a coward, but if you would do that.'

'It is not cowardice to be weak,' said Mma Ramotswe. She stopped herself. That was not quite what she had intended to say, but Mma Makutsi seemed either not to have noticed or not to have taken offence, so Mma Ramotswe left it at that.

Rarely had Mma Ramotswe's life been quite so complicated, but at least she knew what to do about it. The next morning, after sending a message to Mma Makutsi through Mr J. L. B. Matekoni to the effect that she would be in late that day, or perhaps even not at all, she drove her tiny white van along Zebra Drive, out into the traffic of Mobutu Drive, and headed for Mochudi, on the old road. That was the road she knew well, the road she had travelled so many times before, as a child, as a young woman, and now, although still the same person in many respects, as an established and well-known cit-izen, the wife of a much-admired mechanic, the owner of a business with a staff of two and a half (if one counted Mr Polopetsi). Mr Polopetsi . . . It saddened her just to think about it. But that, she supposed, was often the case with anonymous letters: they came from somebody one knew, and when they were signed, as they often were, *A Friend*, that was indeed the case.

But as she drove along the Mochudi road, passing each landmark – that tiny rural school with the stony yard and the crumbling whitewash; that normally dry river course, now with a muddy trickle of water from the previous day's rain; that graveyard just off the road with its tiny shelters, umbrella-like, above each grave, so that the late people down below might be protected from the sun – as she drove along this road with all its memories, she put out of her mind the things that had been worrying her. For out here, out in the acacia scrub that stretched away to those tiny island-like hills on the horizon, the concerns of the working world seemed of little weight. Yes, one had to earn a living; yes, one had to work with people who might have their little ways; yes, the world was not always as one might want it to be: but all of that seemed so small and unimportant under this sky. The important thing, and really the only thing, Mma Ramotswe told herself, is that you are breathing and that you can see Botswana about you; that was the only thing that counted. And any person, no matter how poor he might be, could do that. Any woman might drive her tiny white van along this road and feel the warm breeze on her face. That was the important thing.

And now, coming into Mochudi, the place where she was born, she followed the road that led round the back of the hill which overlooked the village. There was a choice of trees under which to park, and she picked the one that looked the shadiest. Then, without asking herself why she should be here and why she should seek out that place at the edge, where the rock stopped and there was several hundred feet of tumbling noth-ing in front of you, she made her way over to that place and looked down. This was where she had come with Mr J. L. B. Matekoni when he had been recovering from his depressive ill-ness – his sadness as he now called it – and they had sat together. This was where, many years before, she had played with her friends as a child, daring each other to go closer to the edge, risking the ire of the teacher who had banned them from going anywhere near the void. This was where she could sit and hear the sound of the cattle bells drifting up from below. This was where she could always find peace.

She sat, doing nothing, staring out over the plain below. If, when viewed from above like this, our human striving could seem so small, then why did it not appear like that when viewed from ground level? And as she thought this, she allowed her mind to turn to the problems in hand. The question of Mr Polopetsi was the most serious of these, she felt, but here, in this light, he was no problem. If envy had driven him to write what he had written, then there was a very simple remedy for that. Love. She would tell him that she was sorry that he had been hurt into writing those letters. She would promote him. So that solved that.

Then there was Mr J. L. B. Matekoni and his determination to take Motholeli to Johannesburg. Of course it was hopeless: this doctor, whoever he was, had no business raising Mr J. L. B. Matekoni's hopes like that. There was nothing that could be done for Motholeli – that had been made quite clear by the doctors at the Princess Marina when they had done their scan. They had shown her the results and pointed to the place they thought was responsible. They said that if there had been a tumour, which could be operated upon, it would have shown. But there was nothing. A diagnosis by elimination, they explained: there had been damage caused by infection, by something nobody could see. They had been firm in their view that this was the explanation, and so too had they been firm in their view that Motholeli would never walk. That had to be accepted, and this doctor was simply raising hopes that would have to be dashed. And when she had probed, and got Mr J. L. B. Matekoni to admit it, she had uncovered the doctor's motivation: money. Mr J. L. B. Matekoni had not revealed how he would pay, but here, on this rock, payment seemed not to be the issue. Let him do what he wished. If he wanted to take Motholeli to Johannesburg, then he should be allowed to do so. What was the point of striving to stop somebody from doing something when the sky was as large as this and when you could see, on the dry land stretching out below, the first touches of green from the rains?

And Mma Makutsi and her bed? That was simple; hardly a problem at all. She should tell Phuti Radiphuti the truth, because that was what he was owed; but the truth would include the fact that Mma Makutsi was afraid to speak to him about what she had done. Mma Sebina and her lies? Simple too: she must be treated as if she was telling the truth, *because that was what she thought it was.* Everything, in fact, was very clear, and very untroubling. In such a way might worries be lifted, allowing them to float up of their own accord, float up off one's shoulders and disappear into the high sky of Botswana, so empty, so white, that it made one feel dizzy simply to look at it.

She rose to her feet and for a moment felt unsteady. It would be so easy to fall, she thought, to go over the edge in that moment of disorientation that can come when you suddenly stand up and the blood rushes from the head. But the feeling passed, and she was steady enough as she took one last look at the land down below, the piece of this earth that she knew so well. Then she picked her way across the rocks to the place where the tiny white van was parked, got into it, and began the drive back to Gaborone. The landmarks of her journey earlier that day would repeat themselves in the opposite order: graveyard, river bed, whitewashed school, home. The wrong order for a journey, thought Mma Ramotswe, and smiled.

Chapter Ten

The Doctor's House

Mr J. L. B. Matekoni had not told Mma Ramotswe that he had set up an appointment for Motholeli to see the doctor from Selebi-Phikwe. He did not wish to deceive her, but his suspicion that she would not approve had been proved right.

'There is no point,' she said. 'We know that, Rra. We have been told.'

He had rehearsed his arguments to the contrary, and he had used them. There was such a thing as a second opinion, he pointed out; there were plenty of cases in which one doctor had given up and then another doctor had achieved a cure. Were there? she asked. And did he know of anywhere this thing that Motholeli had, this precise thing, had been cured?

He knew that he was no match for Mma Ramotswe; it was something to do with the sort of mind she had, a detective's mind, which would always come up with arguments that he, a mere mechanic, would never be able to refute. But there were second opinions, and he held his ground.

'It's the same with cars,' he argued. 'If you brought a car into the garage and Charlie told you that he thought you needed a new gearbox, wouldn't you want a second opinion? And might not that second opinion be quite different from Charlie's?'

That was a powerful example, as far as it went; but Mma Ramotswe did not think that it went very far. 'Charlie is not a proper mechanic, Mr J. L. B. Matekoni,' she said. 'Nobody would listen to his opinion in the first place.' She paused, letting the point sink in. She was being gentle here, because she knew that he wanted desperately to believe that this doctor could do something. 'Those doctors at the Princess Marina knew what they were doing. And Dr Moffat as well. He said the same thing, too, didn't he? Wouldn't you prefer to listen to Dr Moffat rather than Charlie?'

He had let the matter ride at that, but he was still determined, and the next day he had lifted Motholeli gently into his truck.

'It's best if you don't discuss this with Mma Ramotswe,' he had said to her. 'There is a doctor I would like you to see, but I don't think Mma Ramotswe likes him very much.'

Motholeli had been puzzled. 'Why does she not like him?' she asked. 'Is he unkind?'

Mr J. L. B. Matekoni laughed. 'Of course not! He is a very kind doctor who has said that he will just take a look at your legs to see if there is anything he can do to help. He probably won't be able to do anything, I'm afraid, but I think we should see him, don't you?'

She did. She had become reconciled to being in a wheel-chair, adapting in the way children will adapt to virtually any adversity. This, in her eyes, was how the world was, and she had neither moped nor railed against her illness. At the same time, she still dreamed that she could walk, and these dreams came quite frequently; not day-dreams, but sleeping dreams in which she suddenly slipped out of the wheelchair and simply walked like other children.

'I am happy to see this doctor,' she said. 'I know . . .'

'Yes,' said Mr J. L. B. Matekoni. 'We must not go with any hopes. But we can at least go.'

Now, sitting in the passenger seat of Mr J. L. B. Matekoni's truck, Motholeli gave an anxious glance at her wheelchair, which was in the open back of the vehicle and was bouncing about as the truck negotiated the dirt road which led to the doctor's house.

Mr J. L. B. Matekoni reassured her that it would be safe. 'We are almost there,' he said. 'That is Mr Mgang's house over there, you see, and that means we are only a mile from the doctor's place.'

The road curved round to the right, back in the direction of town. On either side of the road was scrub bush of a neglected and desolate nature, half-heartedly grazed by a small herd of thin cattle, dusty even after the first fall of rain, dotted with stunted acacias and discouraged thorn bushes. The road was now little more than a track, so deeply rutted in the centre that it was safer to drive with the wheels on one side up on the thick verge of sand. A lesser vehicle might quickly be bogged down and sink in this sand, but not Mr J. L. B. Matekoni's truck, with its wide tyres and its low-ratio gears.

The doctor's gate appeared without warning in the fence. Beyond it, another track, but not a very long one, leading to the house itself, which was set down beside a small stand of eucalyptus trees; a house which must once have been a farmhouse, back in the nineteen fifties, in Bechuanaland Protectorate days, before Botswana. Along the front of the house ran a verandah, with squat white-painted pillars supporting a sloping tin roof that had been painted deep red. Here and there, where the weather had made its mark, the paint had worn off and the corrugated surface of the tin below was revealed, rusty patches of discoloration. A single telephone wire ran from the roof of the house to a pole by a water tank, and then to another pole, marching off to join other wires near the side of the road. Oddly, inconsequentially, Mr J. L. B. Matekoni muttered, 'That carried my voice.' And Motholeli, looking up, said, 'What?'

'That telephone wire,' said Mr J. L. B. Matekoni. 'It carried my voice when I phoned the doctor to make your appointment.'

She frowned. 'Yes. And is that him, that man? Is that the doctor?'

He had come out and was watching them from the shade of the verandah, a tall man, his tight greying hair looking almost white against the dark of his skin.

'Where is he from?' asked Motholeli. 'Is he a Motswana?'

'He is half Motswana,' said Mr J. L. B. Matekoni. 'Motswana mother, Zambian father. But he has lived here a long time. He is a very clever doctor, I think. He is called Dr Mwata.'

They parked by the side of the house and Mr J. L. B. Matekoni unloaded the wheelchair from the back. Then he picked up Motholeli and helped her gently into the chair. This is why I am here, he thought; this is why I have come here.

Dr Mwata had emerged from the verandah and was looking down at Motholeli. 'So this is the young lady,' he said.

Mr J. L. B. Matekoni fingered the crease on his trousers. He had changed out of his garage clothes into freshly ironed khaki trousers and a white, short-sleeved shirt. 'She is called Motholeli,' he said. 'She . . .' He tailed off. He was awed by the doctor's presence, which was a powerful one; by his big hands; by the gold-rimmed glasses he wore; and by the fact that he was a man of education, a graduate of a university somewhere, the beneficiary of years of training.

'Come inside,' said the doctor. 'This way.'

Mr J. L. B. Matekoni pushed the wheelchair round to the front of the house and with the help of the doctor lifted it up the three low steps onto the verandah. Then they followed the doctor through the front door and down a short corridor. The floor of the corridor was lined with wide planks which had been recently varnished and reflected the little light that penetrated the gloom of the interior.

'This is a fine house,' said Mr J. L. B. Matekoni nervously.

'It is too old,' said the doctor. 'But it will last me out. Then the white ants will finish their job of eating it. They are waiting for that.'

'They will eat the whole country one day,' said Mr J. L. B. Matekoni. 'They are waiting for us to let them.'

The doctor laughed. 'They do not like the creosote I use,' he said. 'That spoils their appetite.'

He opened a door and led them into a large room furnished with a desk and a few chairs; a bookcase under the window was stuffed with yellowing journals and papers. There was a kitchen table of some sort, raised up by the positioning of bricks beneath its legs so that it was high enough to be an examination couch. A sheet had been draped over this; a sheet with a red line through it signifying hospital ownership.

Suddenly Motholeli started to cry. The doctor became aware of it first and bent down to comfort her. 'You mustn't be frightened,' he said. 'There is nothing to be frightened of.' He turned to Mr J. L. B. Matekoni. 'Perhaps it might have been better if the mother . . .'

'The mother is late. There is just my wife, and she . . .'

The doctor nodded. 'The child will be all right,' he said. And with that he leaned over and lifted Motholeli out of the chair and placed her on the table. She reached out and held on to the sleeve of his shirt. Her head was bent.

'Maybe . . .' began Mr J. L. B. Matekoni. 'Maybe . . .' He did not know what to do. He could not bear her sobbing, which was louder now.

'Hush,' said Dr Mwata. 'There is nothing to cry about. I'm not going to hurt you.'

'No,' said Mr J. L. B. Matekoni. 'This will not hurt.'

Motholeli looked at him. She was trying to stifle her sobs, and was succeeding now.

'There,' said Dr Mwata. 'There, you see.'

He had taken a small rubber hammer out of his pocket and was tapping at her knees. Then he slipped off her shoes and pinched the skin of her ankles. 'Can you feel that?' he asked. 'Or this? Over here? This?'

The examination continued for ten minutes or so. Mr J. L. B. Matekoni looked away, staring out of the window, his back turned so that the doctor might conduct his examination in private. There was an old metal windmill outside, and the wooden blades were turning slowly in the breeze, driving a borehole pump; he could hear the mechanical sucking noise, the rattling of a loose spar on the windmill tower; this was not a well-kept place, but the doctor must be busy, even if he had retired. You could not expect an educated man to worry about pumps and boreholes; there were plenty of other people to attend to such things. In the distance, towards the South African border, the clouds were building up again; there would be more rain, he thought, which was a good sign. Yesterday's storm had laid the dust, and if rain followed later today it would begin to fill the rivers and dams. They could at least hope.

Dr Mwata cleared his throat. 'That is all I need to see,' he said, patting Motholeli on the shoulder. 'You have been a very good girl. Now the Daddy can lift you off the table.'

Mr J. L. B. Matekoni stepped forward and placed the child back in her wheelchair. He was occasionally referred to as the Daddy by people who did not know, but the word remained strange in his ears.

Dr Mwata now took Mr J. L. B. Matekoni's arm. 'You and I should go for a walk, Rra.' He turned to Motholeli. 'I will ask the lady in the kitchen to make you something to drink. She will look after you for a little while. The Daddy and I will not be long.'

He went to the door and called out down the corridor. A few moments later a woman appeared. She was a large woman wearing a housecoat and a pair of commodious blue slippers. She stared at Motholeli while her employer gave instructions. 'You must give this girl some milk. And bread with plenty of honey on it.'

The men went outside, leaving the house from the back door. The yard at the back was neglected too – a patch of land which merged, without fence or marker, into the scrub bush. A few bricks had been placed in the ground in a circle, a forlorn attempt at decoration or the abandoned beginning of a flower bed; apart from that there was nothing.

'This is a nice place,' said Mr J. L. B. Matekoni. He did not know what to say; I am just a mechanic, he thought.

The doctor glanced at him and then looked away. 'We could walk over that way. There is a water tank.' He paused. 'We will have rain later on, I think.'

'I think so too,' said Mr J. L. B. Matekoni. 'Your cattle—'

'They are not mine,' the doctor interrupted him. 'They belong to my son. He is the one who has cattle. I have never had a cattle post. Nothing like that.'

'You are a doctor. You don't have time for that. You have more important things to do.'

The doctor nodded. 'Maybe. But sometimes the things that doctors do may not seem to be all that important. When I was a doctor up on the mines, most of the time I was giving medicals to men before they were signed on. I had to make them run a mile in the heat and then take their pulse. I looked in their mouths for obvious signs of infection, into their eyes, while all the time, you know, the thing that was going to do the real damage was invisible. No microscope would show you it was there. But it was there. And it was years before we knew what it was and what it would do to our people.' He stopped walking and looked at Mr J. L. B. Matekoni. 'Do you know what I'm talking about, Rra?'

Mr J. L. B. Matekoni did not meet his eyes. He looked at the ground. 'I do.'

They had stopped walking while the doctor spoke; now they resumed. 'I lost heart,' said Dr Mwata. 'What could I do? We had the drugs but could we ever get them to people in time? And then they came and said to me that I was too old to carry on. But I did not want to leave medicine altogether. And so I have found a way of helping, particularly those people who have been told by other doctors that nothing can be done. I take on lost causes, you could say. Like that saint. What do they call him? St Jude, I think. The Catholics have this saint who will help them when nobody else will.'

They were nearing the water tank, a low-built, half-crumbling concrete construction to which an old lead pipe ran up from the ground.

'Do you think that you can help her?' asked Mr J. L. B. Matekoni. 'Do you?'

They were at the side of the tank. At the edge of the concrete, where it rose up from the sandy soil, a snake had abandoned its old skin, the slough a gossamer tube, twisted by the wind, but still a perfect mould of the creature that had been within. Dr Mwata reached down and picked it up, delicately holding it so that the sun shone through the crinkle of tiny scales.

'What sort of snake do you think this came from, Mr Matekoni?'

Mr J. L. B. Matekoni shook his head. 'I cannot tell,' he said.

'It is a puff-adder,' said Dr Mwata. 'Look at this bit here – you can tell from that. See?'

Mr J. L. B. Matekoni shuddered. 'I am glad that he is no longer in his skin,' he said.

This remark appeared to amuse Dr Mwata. 'Yes, indeed. I have had to treat people for bites from these,' he said. 'Very nasty. The venom kills tissues. You never fully recover from one of these bites. The muscle around the bite will always be in pretty bad shape. Even with treatment.' He dropped the skin, which floated down to the ground. He looked at Mr J. L. B. Matekoni. 'You ask whether I can do anything. Well, the answer is yes. I think so.'

Mr J. L. B. Matekoni stood quite still. He was aware, though, that the wind had picked up and that the high purple clouds which he had seen in the distance were coming their way. But this was not a time to think about rain; this was a time to think about what the doctor had said. He could help. There was something he could do.

'You can help? You can perform an operation, Rra?'

Dr Mwata shook his head. 'We must get back to the house, Rra. No, I cannot perform an operation, but I do know of a place, a place in Johannesburg, where there are people who work with people who are paralysed. They work with them and see whether they can get the mind to tell the body to move. They could see her and try. I know them. I have sent people to them before and I have had good results.'

'They could walk?'

Dr Mwata hesitated. 'Yes. They were able to walk.'

'And Motholeli?'

'Maybe.' He was silent, licking the tip of a finger and holding it up into the wind. It was the sort of wind that preceded rain; stronger now, cooler. Suddenly he said, 'Do you believe in miracles, Mr Matekoni?'

Mr J. L. B. Matekoni was tongue-tied. Did he believe in miracles? He was not sure. He had seen old engines start when he never thought they would; he had seen cars continue against all the mechanical odds. These were the miracles of the world of mechanics, but there was always a reason, a mechanical reason, to explain them. 'I don't think so,' he said.

The doctor seemed surprised. 'But you want one to happen, don't you?'

Mr J. L. B. Matekoni thought about this. Did he want a miracle to happen? Of course he did. He gave his answer. 'Yes.'

'And do you think miracles are free?' asked Dr Mwata. He spoke quietly, and Mr J. L. B. Matekoni almost did not hear him.

'Yes, surely . . .'

The doctor looked at him, quizzically, and Mr J. L. B. Matekoni realised that this was not the answer that he had expected.

'No. Maybe they aren't free.'

Dr Mwata seemed satisfied with this answer. 'Precisely.'

Mr J. L. B. Matekoni looked up at the sky. He thought that he had felt the first drop of rain, but it could not have been that, as the sky directly above was still clear. 'How much does a miracle cost?' he asked.

'Twenty-five thousand pula,' said Dr Mwata.

Mr J. L. B. Matekoni was aware that Dr Mwata was watching his reaction to this information. The doctor's body, he thought, those long limbs, had become tense. And he noticed, too, that when he said, 'Yes, I shall pay,' the tension disappeared, as if a taut string had suddenly been cut. But this means nothing, he told himself. If there was a chance of a miracle – the remotest chance – he would take it. And was it unreasonable that one should have to pay for a miracle, when all else in this life seemed to cost money, except love, perhaps, which cost nothing, could often be unconditional, and, what was more, made one want to believe in the possibility of miracles?

Chapter Eleven

A Conversation
about the Past

Mma Ramotswe had a living to be earned, of course: more than one, if one took into account Mma Makutsi's salary as an associate detective and the contribution which the agency made to Mr Polopetsi's pay as a part-time helper, mostly in the garage but sometimes in the agency. That could change, thought Mma Ramotswe: if it was true that Mr Polopetsi was the author of the anonymous letters, as she feared he was, he would have to go. Her earlier decision that she might respond to his treachery with love – a solution which had seemed attractive in that moment of peace on the hillside at Mochudi – had been replaced by a more realistic assessment of the situation. She did not relish the thought of dismissing him, but she saw no real alternative. One could not harbour a snake in the bosom of a business, no matter how charitable one felt, and no matter how understanding one was.

But now the immediate task was to attend to a matter that would bring in fees to keep everybody alive. Mma Sebina's case was problematic: she could be lying, but so far Mma Ramotswe only had the word of that strange woman in Otse who claimed to have been present at the birth. Faced with these starkly contradictory testimonies, Mma Ramotswe had decided to work on the assumption that Mma Sebina was telling the truth and that the mother had done so too. Two testimonies to one; simple arithmetic, if nothing else, pointed in that direction. Of course, if she found somebody else who had light to throw on the mystery, then that might tip matters the other way. For all she knew, further inquiries might make the score two all, but time would settle that uncertainty.

At least she had the names of some more of the elder Mma Sebina's friends, and that gave her something to work on. She had set Mma Makutsi to work on the tracing of these people – a task which her assistant always performed quickly and effectively, principally through resort to the Botswana telephone directory, but also through the judicious use of a cousin in the tax office. This cousin was happy to reveal the addresses of taxpayers to Mma Makutsi, whom she had long admired. So when Mma Ramotswe had given her the names of the friends of Mma Sebina's mother, it had taken Mma Makutsi not much more than a day to come up with a neatly typed list of names and addresses. There had been four names on the list; three had been traced, and only one still had a question mark pencilled in against it. Of the three names for which an address had been found, two were in Gaborone: one lived in a flat near the new magistrates' court, the other in a house a few blocks away from the Grand Palm Hotel. Both had telephone numbers.

On the morning after her trip to Mochudi, Mma Ramotswe left the office to seek out the woman who lived near the Grand Palm Hotel. She had had a short discussion with Mma Makutsi before she left, but it had touched only briefly on the Sebina case. Mma Makutsi was more concerned about the ruined bed and the imminent return to town of Phuti Radiphuti.

'He will be back tomorrow, Mma Ramotswe,' she said. 'And the first thing he will ask is: how is the new bed? And what will I say to that? It is no longer? Is that what I will say?'

'We must tell him before he asks,' said Mma Ramotswe. 'And remember, I have offered to do this thing for you. I will go to see him and tell him what happened.'

Mma Makutsi winced. 'Oh, Mma . . .'

Mma Ramotswe smiled. 'For goodness' sake, Mma Makutsi! It is only a bed. There are many beds in this country. There are millions of beds . . .'

She stopped. Were there millions of beds in Botswana? Was that, perhaps, an exaggeration?

Mma Makutsi noticed the hesitation. *Be Accurate* had been the motto of the Botswana Secretarial College, and she could not let this wild statement pass. 'I think that there are less than two million people in this country,' she said. 'And not everyone has a bed. There are some people who have no bed at all, and then there are all those people who share a bed. So there are not millions of beds, Mma Ramotswe. There are maybe . . .'

Charlie had come in at this point, bearing the mug from which he drank his tea. 'Beds?' he said. 'What is all this about beds?'

'We are having a private conversation about beds,' snapped Mma Makutsi. 'This is women's talk. It is none of your business.'

Charlie made a face. 'You and that Phuti man – have you got one bed or two?'

Mma Makutsi's eyes widened in anger. 'That is none of your business!'

'Just asking,' said Charlie.

'You should not ask these personal questions,' said Mma Ramotswe gently. 'It is not polite, Charlie.'

Charlie shrugged. 'Modern people talk about these things quite freely,' he said. 'You ladies must be more up to date.'

Mma Ramotswe shook a finger at him, but playfully. 'You are a naughty boy, Charlie.'

'He is a stupid boy,' muttered Mma Makutsi.

'I am a man,' said Charlie. 'I am not a boy. And anyway, Mma, talking of beds, I saw a bed just like yours the other day. You know, the one that got ruined in the rain. The one with the heart. I saw one on sale. Cheap, cheap. Shop-soiled, I think, but very cheap.'

Mma Makutsi, who had turned to look pointedly away during this exchange, now spun round. Where was this bed, she demanded. And the price? Charlie told her, and she looked thoughtful.

Mma Ramotswe, grasping the situation, shook her head. 'It is better to tell the truth,' she said. 'It is always better, Mma.'

Mma Makutsi pursed her lips. 'Except sometimes,' she muttered.

She spoke so softly that Mma Ramotswe did not hear what she said. And she had things to do before she left to speak to the woman who lived near the Grand Palm Hotel.

There are not enough trees in this part of town, thought Mma Ramotswe, as she searched for somewhere to park her tiny white van. That was the trouble with those new developments: the first thing that builders did when they arrived to start their work was to cut down all the trees. Then, even if they planted new trees, it would take years before there was enough shade to cover a person, let alone a vehicle. Some people resorted to shade netting, which provided shelter from the sun, but ultimately there was nothing to beat the shade provided by a tree; leafy, natural shade that made patterns on the ground.

She settled for the grossly inadequate cover provided by a small thorn tree that had somehow escaped the builders' notice. Then, checking the plot number on the fence against the number on her piece of paper, she pushed open the gate and called out *Ko, Ko*, as was polite, before entering. Of course, these days one might have to walk up the path uninvited and call out again at the door, but Mma Ramotswe preferred to do things in the proper way. And this morning her call resulted in the appearance of a woman at the side door of the house. She was drying her hands on a small towel; caught in the midst of housework. She was much older than Mma Ramotswe – by thirty years or so – and there was a stiffness to her movements as she beckoned her visitor to come up the path.

Mma Ramotswe introduced herself. 'You do not know me, Mma. I am Precious Ramotswe.'

The woman listened attentively, with the manner that older people have with names. She belonged to a Botswana where names meant something, connected people with places, cousins, events; even with cattle.

'Ramotswe? There was an Obed Ramotswe in Mochudi, I think. He . . .'

'Was my father. He is late now. My father.'

The woman lowered her eyes in sympathy. 'I am sorry. He was a good man.'

Mma Ramotswe felt proud, as she always did when somebody remembered her father. Invariably they used the expression *good man*; and he was. He was the best of men.

The woman invited her into the kitchen and moved an old enamelled kettle onto the ring of a stove. 'I will make tea, Mma,' she said. 'Then we can talk. We can talk about your father. He knew my late husband's brother. They were friends.'

'I think I heard your name mentioned, Mma,' said Mma Ramotswe. 'Mapoi. It seemed a bit familiar. That is why. My father and your late brother-in-law.'

'No, he is not late, that one. My husband is late but his brother is not late. He is living down near Lobatse. I never see him because he is scared to travel. He says that buses crash too often, so he stays down there. We get more frightened as we get older, Mma. Or that's what I sometimes think. More and more frightened – of everything.'

Mma Ramotswe nodded. It was true, she thought. But why? Because we had seen so many things go wrong in our lifetime? Would she end up like that; afraid to travel in a bus?

Mma Mapoi gestured to a chair, and Mma Ramotswe accepted the invitation. It was a traditional chair, strung with strips of cured hide threaded through holes bored into the hardwood frame and then criss-crossed to provide a comfortable seat. It was a chair that harked back to a simpler Botswana, to a Botswana of sweet-breathed cattle by the side of the road, of morning air spiced with the smoke of wood fires; who would need more of a chair than that?

'I have come here because I am a detective,' said Mma Ramotswe. 'No, don't be alarmed. I am not a police detective. I am just somebody who finds things out for people.'

'Missing people?' asked Mma Mapoi.

'Yes, Mma. That is exactly what I do. In this case, I am looking for relatives for somebody. There is a woman called Mma Sebina . . .'

'There *was* a Mma Sebina,' Mma Mapoi corrected her. 'She is late, I'm afraid. Sometimes it seems that everyone is late.'

Mma Ramotswe smiled. 'We all become late, sooner or later. But her daughter—'

146

Mma Mapoi clapped her hands together. 'Of course, Mma. I was forgetting her daughter. I have not seen her recently, you see. I was very friendly with her mother. Is the daughter well?'

Mma Ramotswe assured her that the daughter was well. 'But I have to tell you, Mma,' she went on, 'that there is one thing that is bothering her. She thinks that she is not really the daughter of her late mother. She thinks that she is the daughter of another mother.'

Mma Mapoi received this news in silence. She looked at the kettle, which had not yet boiled. Then she looked down at her hands, which were resting, folded, in her lap. Mma Ramotswe's eyes were drawn to the hands and saw the signs of years of hard work: the cracked skin from scrubbing; the scars from the kitchen knife, little nicks; the worn-down nails.

'She is,' said Mma Mapoi eventually.

'She is the daughter of another mother?'

Mma Mapoi lifted her head. 'Yes. Another mother.'

So it is true, thought Mma Ramotswe. Three testimonies to truth; one to falsehood. That woman in Otse, the woman with the chair in the tree, was making things up. Perhaps I should have been readier to discount the tale of one who had a chair in a tree.

'Do you know who that mother was, Mma?'

Mma Mapoi dropped her gaze again. The kettle was now boiling, but she seemed uninterested in it. Mma Ramotswe wondered if she should offer to make the tea, but decided against it. They would wait. She looked at Mma Mapoi. She had not expected her to know, because it seemed that it would

147

be a bit too much to hope for. But obviously she did know; if she did not, she would have said so.

'Do you know her name, Mma?' she prompted. 'Or even where she came from?'

Mma Mapoi cleared her throat. 'I know who that woman was,' she said. 'I did not know her personally, but I knew exactly who she was.'

'I am glad,' said Mma Ramotswe. 'It is important for the younger Mma Sebina to know. When you do not know where you have come from . . .'

Mma Mapoi suddenly rose to her feet to attend to the kettle. She checked herself in a moment of pain; her joints. 'Is it important, Mma? Are you sure that it's important?'

'I think so,' said Mma Ramotswe. 'People who are adopted want to know these days, I think. They used to hide these things, but not now.'

Mma Mapoi poured the hot water into a small brown teapot. The smell of the tea, Tanganda, Mma Ramotswe thought, drifted across the room. It was time, thought Mma Ramotswe; and tea made it easier to talk, much easier.

'But what if there really is something to hide,' said Mma Mapoi, her voice raised unnaturally. 'What then, Mma?'

It will be marriage, thought Mma Ramotswe. The real mother would have been a young girl, perhaps, the father maybe even unknown. That would have been an issue in the past, but not now, not any more. She began to reassure Mma Mapoi that this would probably not disturb Mma Sebina, but the older woman cut her short.

'No, no, Mma. It's not that. No. That is nothing.'

Mma Ramotswe waited.

'It is something very bad, Mma,' said Mma Mapoi. 'I don't know if I should tell you.' She paused. 'If I do, will you tell her? Will you tell the daughter?'

Mma Ramotswe was uncertain how to deal with this. She had been asked by Mma Sebina to find out about her real family and she did not know how she could agree not to pass on any information she came by. And yet, if it was something terrible, then how could she be sure that Mma Sebina would want to know? Mma Ramotswe began to explain to Mma Mapoi about her duty to her client. She could not undertake to keep anything from her; did Mma Mapoi understand? Rather to her surprise, Mma Mapoi said that she did understand; she understood perfectly well.

'I leave it up to you,' Mma Mapoi said. 'You can decide. But do not tell her until you have thought about it very carefully, Mma. You do not want her to be unhappy, do you?'

'No. Of course not.' Mma Ramotswe waited. Mma Mapoi had poured the tea now and was cradling her cup in her hands. Then she looked up at Mma Ramotswe.

'The mother – the real mother – was a very young woman, Mma. She was just sixteen, I think. And she already had one child before she had this girl. Her first-born was a boy. Then she had a daughter.'

Mma Ramotswe nodded her encouragement. 'I see. Two children.'

'Yes, two children. And then . . . then, Mma, this young

woman killed her husband with a hoe. That is what happened.'

Mma Ramotswe had not been prepared for this. Botswana was a peaceful place, and people did not kill their husbands, or not very often. That happened elsewhere, she thought.

Mma Mapoi was watching her intently. 'I can see that you are shocked, Mma,' she said quietly. 'It was a terrible thing. I think that he was a very bad man, that husband – he beat her, I think, and she decided that she had had enough. That sometimes happens.'

Yes, thought Mma Ramotswe, it did. And she understood. There were men who beat women; she had been married to one, to Note Mokoti, all those years ago. Had she stayed with him, might she have ended up disposing of him? It seemed inconceivable, but in a moment of utter desperation anybody, she imagined, might do anything.

Mma Mapoi continued with her story. 'The police came and took her away. She did not deny that she had killed this man and they took her to the High Court in Lobatse. Mma Sebina – the mother – told me all about this. They knew why she had done it and I think that the judge felt sorry for her, but she still had to go to prison. But she became late there after a year, I think – she was ill. And that made those children orphans.'

'Where did they go? Was there a grandmother?'

Mma Mapoi shook her head. 'No. There was nobody. Nobody knew where that woman was from and the late husband's family would have nothing to do with the children of the woman who had killed their son.'

Mma Ramotswe made a sympathetic clicking with her tongue. Without a grandmother, children in that position would be the responsibility of a village – if they had a village.

'So they took them to that place at Tlokweng,' said Mma Mapoi. 'That is where they went. Then Mma Sebina took the girl. She could not take the brother. She could not feed two more mouths, she said.'

Mma Mapoi went on to say something about the cost of food and how difficult it was to feed growing children, with their appetites. Boys were worse than girls, she said, and they always wanted meat, and meat was so expensive these days, unless you had your own chickens, of course . . . But Mma Ramotswe had stopped listening. The orphan farm at Tlokweng; and there was a boy. I've found your brother, she thought.

'Thank you, Mma,' said Mma Ramotswe. 'You have told me something very important. And I don't think we need to tell Mma Sebina about what her mother did. We can keep that a secret, as long as we can tell her that she has a brother.'

Mma Mapoi seemed relieved. 'It would be better that way,' she said. 'My friend never wanted her daughter to know. I am sure of that.'

'Then we can respect her wishes,' said Mma Ramotswe. 'It is always better to respect the wishes of somebody who is late.'

'Oh, yes,' said Mma Mapoi. 'That is much better. Otherwise they might punish us from up there.'

Mma Ramotswe sipped at her tea. 'Possibly,' she said. But there was disbelief in her voice; she did not think that those who were late, or the ancestors themselves, would wish punishment upon us, no matter what our transgressions. It was far more likely that there would be love, falling like rain from above, changing the hearts of the wicked; transforming them.

Chapter Twelve

About a Bed

It was not until the following morning that it became apparent what Mma Makutsi had been up to while Mma Ramotswe had been on her mission to find Mma Mapoi. Mma Ramotswe had forgotten the conversation with Charlie, and the sudden expression of interest on Mma Makutsi's face when he had remarked on the cheapness of the bed he had seen. That attention became something more than interest once Mma Ramotswe had left the office. Mr Polopetsi, who had been sitting idly in the garage, had been called in and left in charge of the agency, while Mma Makutsi prepared to go to the bank.

'Answer the phone, Rra,' he had been instructed. 'Don't do anything. Just answer the phone and take any messages.'

'And if a client comes in? What then? Am I to send that person away? Away to the competition?'

Mma Makutsi had looked at him in astonishment. 'Competition? What competition are you talking about?'

'Somewhere else,' said Mr Polopetsi, waving his hand vaguely in the direction of the window. 'You cannot send customers away. No business can.'

Mma Makutsi knew what he was driving at. Ever since he had been taken on at the garage – and Mma Makutsi regarded Mr Polopetsi as working for Mr J. L. B. Matekoni, and not for Mma Ramotswe – it had been his ambition to have his own clients. But that could not be allowed, or certainly not at this stage, because he could not be trusted to get things right. And there was another reason that, for Mma Makutsi at least, was a very powerful one for keeping Mr Polopetsi in the background. This was the simple fact that the No. 1 Ladies' Detective Agency was, as the name so clearly spelled out, an agency run by *ladies*. Mr Polopetsi, for all his modesty and keenness, was a *man*, and if he were to be given substantial authority could the business still in good faith be called a ladies' detective agency? Mma Makutsi thought not.

'There is no competition, Rra,' she said patiently. 'We are the only detective agency in town. If somebody doesn't want to come to us, then that is just too bad. Their problems will remain unsolved.'

She waited for him to say something, but he did not. 'So I think,' she went on, 'that it's best for you just to take the client's name and explain that the *detectives'* – and she stressed the word *detectives* – 'will be back later on. Make an appointment for anybody to see me tomorrow morning.'

Mr Polopetsi looked at her. 'But would it not be better to arrange an appointment with Mma Ramotswe herself? Why speak to the dog when you can speak to its master?'

Mma Makutsi stiffened. When she responded, her voice was icy. 'I'm not sure that I understand what you're saying, Rra. What is this about dogs?'

'Oh, I wasn't talking about real dogs,' Mr Polopetsi said quickly. 'I was talking about how it's best to go directly to the top. That's what some people think, Mma. I don't, but they do.'

'That may be true, Rra,' said Mma Makutsi, picking up her handbag, 'but we haven't got time to talk about all that now. Just look after the phone, that's all. Please don't start any new cases. Thank you.'

She left the office and walked down to the place where the minibuses stopped. One of them, she knew, went past the bank and after she had done her business there – withdrawing the sum required – she could go on to the shop where Charlie claimed he had seen the bed. It pained her to think that she would have to withdraw almost half of her savings in order to make the purchase, but there was a lot at stake. She could not face Phuti and tell him that her carelessness had ruined the bed he had bought. Nor could she allow Mma

Ramotswe to tell him on her behalf: the effect, she thought, would be much the same. Indeed, it might be worse, as Phuti might think the less of her for not having the courage to tell him herself. No, the simplest thing was surely to buy another bed and store it safely at the agency or in the garage until Phuti could transport it to his house. For the time being she would continue to sleep on her own old and somewhat uncomfortable mattress, until such time as, sanctified by custom and by the marriage laws of the Republic of Botswana, they sank into connubial bliss in a luxurious and commodious bed, under the protection of a large, heart-shaped headboard in red velvet.

That was what Mma Makutsi had done. The next morning, shortly after nine, while Mma Ramotswe was dictating a letter, Charlie knocked on the door and announced that a delivery van had arrived.

'It's for you,' he said, looking at Mma Makutsi and pointing a greasy finger in her direction. 'It's a you-know-what!'

Mma Makutsi, flustered, looked down at her dictation note-book. Her pencil dropped to the floor.

'That sounds very exciting, Mma Makutsi,' said Mma Ramotswe. 'Perhaps somebody has sent you a present.'

'No,' said Charlie, shaking his head. 'It's a new bed. Just like the other one. She bought it. It's not a present.'

Mma Ramotswe half rose to her feet to look out of the window but stopped herself and sat down again. It was not her business to criticise Mma Makutsi for buying a bed, or anything for that matter. There had been that business with her new blue shoes not all that long ago, when Mma Makutsi had purchased a totally unsuitable pair of new shoes *against* the specific advice of Mma Ramotswe, and where had that led? To disaster. We must remember, Mma, she had said to her assistant as they stood before that tempting shop window, we must remember that those of us with traditionally built feet need to buy traditionally built shoes. It had been good advice; for Mma Makutsi, although by no means as traditionally built as Mma Ramotswe herself, was none the less heading in that direction and would, when older, be of convincingly traditional build. But leaving that to one side, her feet were every bit size eight and these shoes, intended as they had been for some region of Italy where feet were small and slender, were, at the most, size six and a half. Mma Ramotswe's advice on that occasion had been ignored, with the result that there had been a full day in which Mma Makutsi had suffered from considerable discomfort and disability. Indeed, those shoes had turned her head, thought Mma Ramotswe; to the extent that she had even resigned her job – on a temporary basis, as it turned out.

No, Mma Ramotswe would not interfere with any purchase that Mma Makutsi made. And as she merely sat down and said, 'A bed. Well, that will be very useful, Mma,' the thought crossed her mind that perhaps the bed would be too small, just as the shoes had been. But she was not sure whether it was fashionable to have a bed that was too short and narrow; anything was possible in fashion, of course, as fashion and comfort, thought Mma Ramotswe, were inevitably mutually exclusive.

Mma Makutsi now affected nonchalance. 'Yes, Mma. It will. I thought that I would get a new one, to replace the one that I . . . that I left out in the rain. Charlie was right: they were selling them very cheaply and I bought it . . .' Her words tailed off at the end, as if she was suddenly choking with emotion at the thought of what she had done. Half her savings. Half.

Mma Ramotswe sensed Mma Makutsi's discomfort, and understood the reason. 'Don't worry about it, Mma. There are times when we have to buy very expensive things. It is always worthwhile. Always.' It was not, but out of kindness she said that it was.

'Yes,' said Charlie. 'Get the well-known things. Go for the label every time.'

In normal circumstances, Mma Ramotswe would have felt obliged to refute this false philosophy, but not now. 'Charlie,' she said, 'why don't you go and ask those men to put the bed safely in the garage? Just outside that door. It will be safe there.'

Mma Makutsi looked up in gratitude. 'I won't have to keep it there long, Mma,' she said. 'Phuti will come and collect it in a few days.'

'Of course he will,' said Mma Ramotswe reassuringly. 'In the meantime, you will get pleasure from seeing your fine purchase and thinking of how much money you saved – since it was a bargain. That's the important thing. That will make you feel better.'

It did, immediately, and dictation was resumed. They had several letters to complete and a client was coming in half an hour. There would probably not even be time for tea before the client's arrival, but the kettle could be put on once the client had arrived. People talked very freely and comfortably against the sound of a boiling kettle, Mma Ramotswe had found. And they talked even more willingly once they had been served a cup of tea, and the first sips had been taken, warming those regions of the heart that were burdened, that wanted to talk.

The client's problem, as it turned out, was very straightforward – a matter of a tenancy agreement in which the tenant had been substituted in spite of a term in the contract that this should not happen. The owner of the house had not met the original tenant, since she had been away when the original agreement was drawn up by her attorney. Now she had returned and wanted the house back. She had been reconciled to having to let the lease run for another year, but then a neighbour had let drop a nugget of information. 'Your tenant,' she had said, 'says that he is called Moganana. You think he is called that too. But I think that he is the brother-in-law of that Moganana, and that he works over at one of those businesses on the Francistown Road. I can show you the place.'

Mma Makutsi had drawn in her breath audibly at the deception. 'That is cheating,' she muttered.

The client was pleased to find her own outrage endorsed; she did not like the thought that some people might find her selfish for wanting the tenant out. 'You're very right, Mma,' she said, looking over her shoulder at Mma Makutsi. 'That is why I am keen to get this worthless person out of the house. I cannot have a cheat under my roof.'

We all need somewhere to live, thought Mma Ramotswe; but did not say it.

'It will be easy enough to find out,' she said. 'I will follow this person, this person who is not Moganana, from the house in the morning. We shall see where he goes to work. Then it will be easy.' She paused. One would not want the client to imagine that it was too easy, or one's entirely reasonable fee might be resented. 'Or a bit easy,' she added. 'In fact, difficult in parts and easy in others. Quite difficult, though.'

The client, however, was satisfied. 'I'm sure that you will do it well, Mma Ramotswe,' she said. 'And then justice will again reign supreme.'

It was a rather impressive way of describing the hoped-for outcome, but Mma Ramotswe nodded in agreement. People should not lie about who they are, she thought. Even if they do need somewhere to live.

The client looked at her watch. 'I must not stay long, Mma,' she said. 'The tea, though, is very good.'

'It is red bush,' said Mma Ramotswe. 'It comes from down there somewhere.' She pointed south. 'They make it down there and they bring it up here.'

'I see,' said the client. She looked at her watch again. 'Will you do this thing tomorrow? Will you follow that man very soon?'

'I will do it as soon as I can,' said Mma Ramotswe. 'Give us a week to find all this out.'

There was always that moment after the client had left, when Mma Ramotswe and Mma Makutsi looked at one another and reached a view. Sometimes, after a difficult session, they looked at one another in sympathy and embarrassment; on other occasions, the client would barely have left the office before Mma Makutsi would start to giggle. On this occasion there was no such reaction.

'I would like to work on this, Mma,' said Mma Makutsi. 'I feel very sympathetic towards that lady.'

Mma Ramotswe nodded. 'She is entitled to her house,' she said. 'If you let a house to one person another person should not come and live in it. That is definitely dishonest.' She paused for a moment. 'But the problem is, Mma, that you would need to follow that person, and you do not drive. If he works out on the Francistown Road then he probably has a car.'

Mma Makutsi thought for a moment. 'Phuti could drive me,' she said. 'Phuti has offered. He said that any time I needed to be driven anywhere, he would do it. Or he has drivers at the furniture store. He said that one of those men could be sent to drive me.'

Mma Ramotswe considered the offer. She still had to sort out the Mma Sebina matter and it would be useful to delegate something to Mma Makutsi. It would also keep her assistant happy, which was a major consideration, since she would be in a position to leave once she married Phuti

Radiphuti, and Mma Ramotswe did not want that – Mma Makutsi's departure, that is. She was completely in favour of the marriage, of course, as Phuti Radiphuti was a very good man and . . . well, he was good for Mma Makutsi. Or so she thought; but Mma Makutsi herself had suddenly become agitated. She had seen something out of the window; Charlie, perhaps, was up to something. But it was not that. Phuti Radiphuti himself had arrived; as often happens, Mma Ramotswe thought, when we bring people to mind. We bring them to mind and then they turn up in the flesh, or telephone, or do something to remind us that we should be careful of what we think of in this life.

'Phuti!' exclaimed Mma Makutsi, when she saw her fiancé's car, with its distinctive red stripe along the side, drawing up in front of the garage.

'Oh, yes,' said Mma Ramotswe. 'He is back. That's nice for you, Mma. You can ask him about driving you.'

As she spoke, it occurred to her that Phuti's car was not very well suited to detective work, as it was impossible to miss a white car which had a curious red stripe on its side. She had assumed that this was the livery of the Double Comfort Furniture Shop, but had been told that it was not, that Phuti himself had painted it as a decoration. But whatever the origin of the stripe, it was a very noticeable feature and people being followed by a car with a red stripe would probably notice the fact. And Clovis Andersen, she thought, author of *The Principles of Private Detection*, would undoubtedly agree.

This line of thought, though, was interrupted by Mma Makutsi, who was clearly agitated by the unexpected arrival. 'He'll see the bed,' she hissed. 'He'll see it!'

'But he has to,' said Mma Ramotswe. 'Just tell him. Tell him what happened.'

'Tell him?'

Mma Ramotswe was calm. 'Yes, or I will, if you like. I promised you that I would tell him about the other bed. I'm still happy to do that. It will not be hard for me.'

'No,' said Mma Makutsi, her voice full of alarm. 'We cannot do that, Mma. We cannot give Phuti a shock.'

'Nonsense,' said Mma Ramotswe. 'It will not be a shock. Look, here he comes. I'll tell him.'

'No,' implored Mma Makutsi. 'Please, Mma. Leave it. Leave it.'

Mma Ramotswe was silenced. There was no mistaking the passion, and urgency, in Mma Makutsi's words. She would not say anything in those circumstances, but she wondered how Mma Makutsi would explain the new bed. Some explanation would be required – it must be – as Phuti could not but see the bed as he came into the office. It was all very strange.

The door opened, tentatively. Just like Mr Polopetsi, Phuti Radiphuti was not one to barge into a room, and certainly not without the necessary *Ko, Ko.*

Phuti appeared, and greeted Mma Ramotswe politely before turning to smile at his fiancée.

'I was passing by,' he said. 'I don't want to disturb you. You ladies are always so busy.'

'But we always have time for you, Rra,' said Mma Ramotswe. 'You have been up in Serowe?'

Phuti nodded. 'We do business with a store up there. They sell our chairs and—' He broke off and turned to Mma Makutsi. 'I see it has arrived, Grace. The new bed has been delivered here rather than to your house. Is that all right with Mma Ramotswe and Mr J. L. B. Matekoni? Maybe they don't want our new bed cluttering up their place.'

'They don't mind at all,' said Mma Makutsi hurriedly. 'That is fine, Phuti.'

Phuti frowned. 'I thought that they were going to deliver it to your house,' he said. 'Sometimes these people can't get things straight. A simple request like that and they get all mixed up.'

Mma Makutsi said nothing. Across her desk, Mma Ramotswe looked at her assistant. If Mma Makutsi remained silent now, then she would be deliberately misleading Phuti. It would be as bad as telling a direct lie; there could be no other way of looking at it.

The silence continued. Outside, on the branches of the acacia tree, a grey lourie, the go-away bird, fluttered its wings, and Phuti, distracted, looked out of the window. 'That tree always has birds in it,' he said. 'Whenever I come here there are birds.'

Mma Makutsi would have to speak now, thought Mma Ramotswe.

'Yes,' said Mma Makutsi. 'Birds.'

There was a further silence. Then Mma Ramotswe rose

from her chair. 'I shall make you some tea, Rra,' she said. 'After that drive down from Serowe, you must be ready for tea.'

The moment to discuss the bed had passed. The seed of the lie, contained in the first tiny hesitation on Mma Makutsi's part, had sprouted quickly, like a ground vine suddenly sending out its shoots after the first rain. So untruth grows, thought Mma Ramotswe; so easily, so easily. She looked at her assistant as she made her way towards the kettle, but Mma Makutsi looked away.

Chapter Thirteen

The Wedding
of the Baboons

Mma Ramotswe had her misgivings, and these were pro-found – but they were not expressed. She could have pointed out to Mr J. L. B. Matekoni yet again that medical opinion had been united, and unequivocal. Much as everybody wanted Motholeli to be cured of her disability, that was simply not going to happen. Dr Moffat had spelled it out for them, gently, of course, but very clearly, confirming the diagnosis that had been reached in the Princess Marina Hospital. It might have been hard for Mr J. L. B. Matekoni to accept – Mma Ramotswe understood that – but it would have been better for him to do that rather than to harbour hope that really should not be there at all.

Ever since his meeting with Dr Mwata, Mr J. L. B. Matekoni had seemed preoccupied. He had told Mma Ramotswe roughly what had transpired at the consultation, but he had not gone into any detail. In response to her questions as to what precise treatment the doctor had mentioned, he had merely pointed in the direction of the border and said that there was a clinic in Johannesburg where they tackled these things. 'With success,' he added.

'And who will go with her?' asked Mma Ramotswe. It would be difficult for her to leave the business, but she doubted if Mr J. L. B. Matekoni had thought of that. He was a considerate man, and a kind one, but, like many men, his head was filled with details of gearboxes and driveshafts and the like.

He did not take long to answer. 'I shall go,' he said simply. 'I have made arrangements.'

'You will drive over there in your truck?'

He nodded gravely. 'That is all planned. It is five hours to Johannesburg in a truck.' He looked at her, almost reproachfully, as if he imagined that she was trying to sabotage the venture. 'The doctor said that we would be away for about a week to begin with. We might have to go back.'

'If it doesn't work?'

Mr J. L. B. Matekoni gazed out of the window; there was still that air of preoccupation. 'Maybe. He didn't put it that way.'

He pulled himself together. 'Anyway,' he continued. 'While I am away the garage will be looked after by Charlie. I have spoken to him about it. He is quite happy to be in charge.'

Mma Ramotswe caught her breath. 'Charlie?'

Mr J. L. B. Matekoni sighed. 'He will have to learn how to be in charge. When he finishes his apprenticeship, he could be in charge of a whole workshop himself. I have to give him some experience.'

Mma Ramotswe said nothing. She agreed that Charlie should be given experience – in theory, at least – but she could not imagine him being in charge of the garage.

She would be tactful. 'Are you sure? Charlie hasn't finished his apprenticeship yet . . .' And would never finish it, she thought.

Mr J. L. B. Matekoni now showed a rare degree of determination. 'It's all arranged,' he said. 'We shall go tomorrow.'

And now, packing Motholeli's suitcase for the trip to Johannesburg, she found herself folding the young girl's clothes, wondering what would be necessary for whatever lay ahead. Would she spend the time at the clinic in bed? In which case more than two nightgowns would be necessary – the one with flowers on it, the one she liked, and the plain blue one which she liked rather less. And the stiff brush with which she liked to tease out the tight curls of her hair, not that Mma Ramotswe approved of that; braiding would have been better. And the Setswana Bible that she had been given by Mma Potokwani when she had left the orphan farm, which had become a memento of that part of her life, now some years away; of the childhood, really, that had been so hard and empty of love until her arrival, with Puso, at the orphan farm.

That Bible was a talisman, in a way, and she kept it prominently on the table in her room, alongside a piece of deep-blue crystalline rock from the north of Botswana, a piece of a country that was predominantly composed of browns and yellows but had these veins of startling green and blue just beneath the skin of the land.

Motholeli herself seemed to be taking the trip in her stride. Mma Ramotswe had been concerned that her hopes would be raised unnecessarily – indeed that was one of her grounds of objection to the whole idea – but the girl herself was calm.

'You do know what the doctors have told us?' Mma Ramotswe said. 'They always try to help, but sometimes . . .'

She faltered. It was not easy to explain the hard side of things to a child, or to anybody really. Mma Ramotswe would have wished the world to be otherwise, but it was not. She would have wished for the suffering of Africa to be relieved, to be legislated out of existence, but it seemed that this would never be, for fundamental unfairness seemed to be a condition of human life. There were rich, there were poor; and whilst one might rail against the injustices which kept people poor, it seemed that these were stubborn to the point of entrenchment. And in the meantime, whilst waiting for justice, or just for a chance, what could one say to the poor, who only had one life, one brief spell of time, and were spending their short moment of life in hardship? And what could she say to Motholeli?

Children are resilient. 'I know, Mma,' said Motholeli. 'I know that the doctors have said they cannot help me. I do not

mind if this new doctor tries. Maybe there are clever doctors
in Johannesburg who can do this thing. But I will not mind if
they cannot.'

Mma Ramotswe reached out and took her hand. 'You are a
brave girl. I am very proud of you.'

The next morning, Mma Ramotswe awoke early, before the
sun had risen, but at that point when the sky was beginning to
go from the dark velvet of night to the lighter cobalt of day.
Mr J. L. B. Matekoni was still asleep, and she shook his shoulder; he was a deep sleeper and would be impervious to an
alarm clock or a lesser touch than this.

'I will make you tea, Rra,' she said. 'I will bring it to you in
bed, and then you can get up and have a good breakfast. You
have a long drive ahead of you.'

He grunted his acknowledgement, and she moved
through to the kitchen. Light under a door had told her that
Motholeli was already awake; she would get herself out of bed
and dressed without any prodding from Mma Ramotswe. She
was like that, even on a normal day, whereas her brother,
Puso, resisted every imprecation to stir, and would hide under
the blanket rather than emerge one minute earlier than
absolutely necessary. Such contrasts, thought Mma
Ramotswe, in two children who are from the same mother
and father; recipes of the blood differed so much, made one
lazy and another energetic, made one like pumpkin and
another like beans; made one – like Mma Makutsi – method-
ical and good at filing, and another – like Charlie – slipshod

and untidy. Not, of course, that Charlie and Mma Makutsi were brother and sister; they had crossed her mind merely as types.

Charlie and Mma Makutsi as brother and sister: the delicious thought begged to be explored. What if such a relationship were to be discovered, through some long-ignored error in the maternity hospital, or through the confession of some wicked midwife who had switched babies? Would Mma Makutsi, who had often said after the death of her poor brother, Richard, that she would relish the thought of another brother, accept Charlie as that new brother? Or would she feel about him in exactly the same way as she felt about him now, unrelated? And as for Charlie, would he in such circumstances regret that he had once famously called Mma Makutsi a warthog? For that, surely, would make him the brother of a warthog, and therefore a warthog himself! We should be careful, thought Mma Ramotswe, of the insults we fling at others, lest they return and land at our own feet, newly minted to apply to those who had first coined them.

Such thoughts reminded Mma Ramotswe that she was now dealing with precisely such a matter, or would be dealing with it, when she got back to the Mma Sebina case. So, as she stood at the gate and waved goodbye to Mr J. L. B. Matekoni and Motholeli as they set off on their journey to the clinic over the border in Johannesburg, she was thinking not only of the little girl, hunched so poignantly in the passenger seat of the cab, but also of the inquiry which she would make later that morning in the office of her friend Mma Potokwani,

tireless defender of orphans, maker of the finest fruit cake in
Botswana, or at least in their part of Botswana, and custodian,
she hoped, of a secret that would bring great joy to Mma
Sebina. That is, if her brother really was going to be a joy;
some brothers were not. But let us just assume, she told herself, that this one will be.

'Ah, Mma Ramotswe,' called Mma Potokwani, from the
window of her office at the orphan farm. 'Come inside. Come
over here.'

And as Mma Ramotswe mounted the two low steps that led
up to Mma Potokwani's room, the matron, standing at the
open door, remarked to her guest, 'I can always tell that it is
you, even before I see you. I hear that noise that your van
makes and I know that it is you.'

'What noise does my van make?'

Mma Potokwani held her guest's gaze. Mma Ramotswe
was her friend – an old friend, moreover, and there were not
many subjects one could not raise with an old friend. But
there were some. One thing one should never do is to criticise, even in the gentlest of manners, the spouse of a friend;
nor their children; nor their taste in music, their dogs, their
possessions in general, their choice of clothes in particular,
their children's choice of clothes (or spouses), or their cook-
ing. Apart from that, one could talk about anything.

But could she talk to Mma Ramotswe about the noise that
her tiny white van was undoubtedly making? The problem
here, thought Mma Potokwani, might be one of simple

denial; people denied things, pretended that they did not exist; wished noises, and other things, out of existence. Mr J. L. B. Matekoni had confessed to the matron that he thought it was high time that Mma Ramotswe got rid of the van and bought a more modern and indeed more commodious vehicle – one more suited to a person of her standing in society, which was, of course, that of the owner of a small, but nonetheless moderately successful, business. Mma Potokwani had agreed with this view, but had expressed the reservation that Mma Ramotswe appeared inordinately attached to her tiny white van and might be difficult to prise out of the driver's seat. She had intended this as a metaphor, but that did not stop her imagining a scene in which a struggling Mma Ramotswe, tenaciously hanging on to the steering wheel, was being pried out of the seat by Mr J. L. B. Matekoni and Charlie, both wielding one of those levers that they used to take tyres off the wheels of cars.

Mma Potokwani decided that she could – indeed should – mention the noise. Friendship required this, if nothing else did. After all, we might not hear the noises made by our own cars, since we generally travelled away from them, leaving them to be heard by those behind us. And if friends did not refer to the fact that one was making a noise, then who would? At this point Mma Potokwani remembered the delicate situation she had found herself in when she had felt herself obliged to draw the attention of one of the orphan farm housemothers to the fact that her stomach was constantly making noises which, on occasion, frightened the smaller children. That had been a delicate interview in which the subject of diet had been raised; beans, suggested Mma Potokwani, were not the ideal food for one in that position and perhaps the house-mother should try eating something less voluble. That had led to an icy silence, ended only by the housemother's stomach.

'It's a sort of rattle,' said Mma Potokwani. 'Or shall I say it's a knocking sound. Like this.' She tapped on the surface of her desk.

'But that is the sound that any engine makes,' said Mma Ramotswe.

Mma Potokwani smiled. 'I don't think so, Mma. Engines normally go like this . . .' and here she imitated an engine. 'That is how they go, Mma. They do not make a knocking sound . . .' she paused, and then concluded, 'unless there is something wrong.'

For a while nothing was said, either by Mma Ramotswe or by Mma Potokwani. Through the window in the office, the same window through which Mma Potokwani had shouted her welcome, came the sound of children singing. Mma Ramotswe tried to make out the words of the song; it was one of those tunes one knew but did not know, and for a moment she put Mma Potokwani's comment out of her mind.

'Such a funny little song, that,' said Mma Ramotswe, her head tilted to the side, as if the better to catch the words as they drifted in. 'About the baboons. Yes, it is. I remember it now.'

'It is about the wedding of the baboons,' said Mma Potokwani. 'It's about what the baboons were wearing to their wedding. What the guests were wearing too. A pair of overalls and an old maternity dress.'

Mma Ramotswe laughed. She was trying to remember when she had heard that song last; it must have been when she was a girl, quite a small girl, in Mochudi. The aunt of one of her friends had sung those songs, and they had sat at her feet. It was so long ago and she could not remember any of the details; the face of the aunt was a blur, and even her recollection of her friend herself was hazy. But there was warmth, and sun, the memory of sun; and the aunt's voice came back to her like the sound of a scratchy old recording of the sort that they played on Radio Botswana when they were talking about things that had happened a long time ago, the voices of old chiefs discussing the things that were important then but now were nothing very much.

From laughter to tears; it happened so quickly, and inexplicably; just those memories were enough. Mma Potokwani immediately sprang to her feet. 'Mma Ramotswe. Mma Ramotswe. I am sorry, Mma. I am very sorry.' She had not imagined that there would be tears for that old white van, but she must love it; of course she loves it, and oh, I am a very tactless person, thought Mma Potokwani. This is my friend and I tell her that her van is dying. I am a very tactless person indeed.

'I should not have said that about your van,' she said, moving over to place her arm round Mma Ramotswe's shoulder. 'Even if it is making a noise – and it is not a very loud noise – it can surely be fixed. You're married to the best mechanic in Botswana by far. By far, Mma. If anybody can fix that van, then it is Mr J. L. B. Matekoni.'

Mma Ramotswe wiped at her eyes with the back of her hand. 'I am the one who should say sorry, Mma. I have come to your office and I am crying. I am sorry.'

'Your van will be fine,' said Mma Potokwani soothingly.

'But it is not my van,' said Mma Ramotswe. 'It is because I was remembering some things. That song that the children were singing – the one about the wedding of the baboons – made me cry. I was remembering how I heard it when I was in Mochudi, a long time ago, when my daddy was still alive. And I thought that all that was gone now. That Mochudi. That lady who sang the song.' She paused, and looked up at Mma Potokwani. 'Sometimes I feel that our whole country has gone, Mma.'

Mma Potokwani thought about this for a moment. Then she shook her head. 'No, it has not gone, Mma. Some of it, maybe. But not the heart that beats right inside the country. Right inside. That is still there.'

'And I feel so sorry for the baboons,' said Mma Ramotswe. 'I know that it is silly to say that. But I suddenly felt very sorry for them. They are just baboons, but they are dressing up for the wedding. Why is that so sad, Mma?'

'Because it is always sad when people try to do things that they cannot do,' said Mma Potokwani. 'The baboons are very sad for that reason.'

They sat in silence for a few minutes. Then Mma Potokwani asked, 'Are you feeling better now, Mma Ramotswe?'

And Mma Ramotswe replied, 'Yes, I am, Mma. That was silly of me.'

Mma Potokwani evidently did not agree. 'No, it was not, Mma Ramotswe. Sometimes I sit here and I think about things. I think about the stories of these children and what some of them have seen in their short lives. And then I find myself crying a bit, Mma. Nobody sees me, but I cry too. The children think, and the housemothers too, they all think: oh, that matron, that Mma Potokwani, she is very strong. But they do not know. They do not know, Mma.'

Mma Ramotswe nodded. Mma Potokwani was right. We all had our moments, and they could descend at any time. It was not just the baboons and their wedding, she thought; it was everything: Motholeli going off to Johannesburg, to face inevitable disappointment; the troubles of Mma Makutsi; Charlie; everything, really. Sometimes everything could just seem too much.

'I have some fruit cake,' said Mma Potokwani suddenly. 'I think that fruit cake is often very good on these occasions.'

'Yes, Mma,' said Mma Ramotswe. 'Yes, you are right. It is.' Fruit cake and tea; sometimes more powerful, in such circumstances, than any words of comfort could be.

Mma Potokwani listened intently as Mma Ramotswe began to tell her of Mma Sebina and her search. Normally she would interrupt Mma Ramotswe as she spoke, not with any rude intent, but merely because she had thought of something that she imagined Mma Ramotswe would like to know and needed to speak about it before it went out of her head; with so much to deal with, constant demands from children and never-ending requests from housemothers, Mma Potokwani had a lot on her mind, and things could easily slip out of it. On this occasion, though, she simply listened, allowing Mma Ramotswe to give an account of her trip to Otse, her meeting with the woman who kept a chair in a tree, and the break-through conversation with Mma Mapoi.

At first Mma Potokwani said nothing when Mma Ramotswe finished. One of the young women who worked in the kitchen had brought in a pot of tea and a plate of cake, and now Mma Potokwani reached forward to pour them each a cup of tea. 'We must not let the tea get cold,' she said, passing a cup to Mma Ramotswe. 'There is nothing worse than being given cold tea. Do you know, Mma Ramotswe, I have heard that in America they even drink it with ice. Have you heard that?'

Mma Ramotswe nodded sadly. 'I have, Mma. At first I could not believe it, then somebody told me that it was true. It is a very serious thing.' She paused, throwing a discreet glance at the untouched fruit cake.

Mma Potokwani understood. 'We must not forget the fruit cake,' she said, slipping a slice onto a plate and passing it to her guest. 'That is another thing I have heard. I have been told that some people these days have stopped eating fruit cake. Have you heard that?'

Mma Ramotswe popped half of the fruit cake into her mouth. It was very good. 'No,' she mumbled. 'I have not heard that rumour.'

'Not Mr J. L. B. Matekoni, of course,' Mma Potokwani continued. 'He would never give up fruit cake, would he, Mma?'

Mma Ramotswe smiled. 'I think that Mr J. L. B. Matekoni would do anything for a piece of your fruit cake, Mma Potokwani.'

'That is good to hear,' said Mma Potokwani, 'because we have a small mechanical problem at the moment with the automatic irrigation system for the vegetables. If you wouldn't mind, Mma . . .'

'I shall mention it to him,' said Mma Ramotswe. 'But I was wondering, Mma, what you made of what Mma Mapoi said to me. About those two children and their mother who became late in prison?'

Mma Potokwani reached for the teapot. 'I remember them well,' she said. 'It was shortly after I came here. I was deputy matron then. I only became matron five or six years later.'

'And the children?' Mma Ramotswe pressed. 'What about those two children?'

'Well,' said Mma Potokwani, 'as you know, the girl went down to that lady in Otse. I do not remember her name, but it will be that Mma Sebina. That must be right. I am glad to hear that the daughter is doing well.'

Mma Ramotswe hesitated. She was so close now to the object of her search that she hardly dared ask the question, fearing a disappointing answer. Things happened to people in this life. They went away. Became late. Disappeared. 'And the boy? The brother of that girl?'

Mma Ramotswe knew immediately that the answer was going to be a positive one. You can always read the signs, she thought; the clues are there, and you only have to be moderately observant to notice them.

Mma Potokwani reached for the teapot again; their third cup. 'The boy? Yes, I saw him the other day.' She poured the tea. 'I bump into him from time to time in the bank. The Standard Bank. That is where he works, you see.'

'Still? He's there now?'

Mma Potokwani shrugged. 'Unless he's at another branch. They move them around, I think. But that man always seems to be there. He is quite senior now. He is a sort of deputy-assistant-under-manager, or something like that. You know how they give themselves long titles. I'm just *matron* but in these big offices they have very big titles.'

Mma Ramotswe thought of Mma Makutsi and her desire to be have an impressive-sounding title. And why should people not be allowed a little boost like that, if it made them feel a bit better about themselves? Mma Potokwani should be allowed to call herself matron-general if she liked; in fact, Mma Ramotswe thought, it would rather suit her.

'Can you tell me the name of this man?' she asked. Even if she did not get this information out of Mma Potokwani, she would be able to find him now. But a name would be useful.

Mma Potokwani closed her eyes for a moment. 'I know it, Mma. I know it. Se . . . something or other. Se . . . Sekape. That's it. Sekape. I think that was the name. It is not the name that they came here with, but it is the same man.'

They talked for another half an hour before Mma Ramotswe left. Now that she had the information she needed, Mma Ramotswe was able to relax and enjoy the conversation, which covered a wide range of topics. One of the house-mothers had been unwell and had undergone an operation. The operation had been successful and the details were given. Mma Ramotswe mentioned that she knew somebody who had benefited from a similar operation and was now the manager of a large café. Mma Potokwani nodded. Operations could set one up very nicely – in some cases.

Charlie was mentioned. 'Mr J. L. B. Matekoni is too soft with those boys,' said Mma Potokwani. 'He is too kind.'

'He has always been a kind man,' said Mma Ramotswe. 'That is what he is like. And Charlie will turn out all right in the end.' Then she added, 'I do not know when the end will be, though.'

The subject of Bishop Mwamba was raised. The bishop had been to visit the orphan farm and the children had sung very nicely for him, Mma Potokwani reported. Mma Ramotswe replied that she had heard him give a sermon in the Anglican cathedral that had been very impressive and that even Mr J. L. B. Matekoni, who was known to sleep through sermons, had remained awake.

Then Mma Ramotswe left. As she drove away, she listened carefully to the noise that her van made. It was difficult to tell, as the road was bumpy and cars always squeaked and protested on bumpy roads, but she thought that she could hear it. It was, as Mma Potokwani had suggested, a knocking sound.

For a moment she imagined that the engine was sending her a signal, as prisoners will knock on the wall of a cell to make contact with unseen others. But what was the tiny white van trying to tell her with its knocking? That it was tired? That it had had enough?

Chapter Fourteen

In the Colour of the National Flag

Mma Ramotswe could not contain herself, but had to. The moment she arrived back at the office after her meeting with Mma Potokwani, she picked up the telephone and dialled Mma Sebina's number. All the way back from the orphan farm she had wondered whether she should tell her on the telephone, and had decided that it would be better for her to meet her client and give her the news in person, face to face; there were, after all, delicate aspects to this case. Although the news of her brother's existence, right here in Gaborone, was undoubtedly good news, there was also the issue of the mother and her unfortunate fate. She had told Mma Mapoi that the daughter need not know

what had happened to the mother, and that she would not raise
it with her. But what if she asked? Mma Ramotswe was not sure
whether it would be right to keep this knowledge from her, even
though it might be difficult for her to accept that her mother
had been sent to prison and had died there. And how much
more difficult would it be to accept the reason for her having
been sent to prison in the first place? All of that, thought Mma
Ramotswe, would have to be handled tactfully.

The telephone call was a disappointment. Another voice
answered and informed Mma Ramotswe that she was a neighbour of Mma Sebina and was looking after the house while
Mma Sebina was up in Maun on business. She would be back,
Mma Ramotswe was told, in a couple of days and yes, Mma
Ramotswe could certainly see her there if she came round to
the house before she left for work in the morning.

'And are you the same Mma Ramotswe who has that detective agency on the Tlokweng Road?' asked the voice. 'Are you
that lady, Mma?'

Mma Ramotswe confessed that she was.

'Do you know where that man who built new roofs is?' the
voice went on. 'The one who built three new roofs round
here – all of which let in the rain when it rained so hard the
other day? Can you answer that for me, Mma?'

Mma Ramotswe was patient. 'I do not know everything,
Mma,' she said. 'Did your roof—'

'It did,' said the voice. 'The rain came in everywhere. The
holes in the corrugated iron were too big for the bolts. So the
rain came straight in.'

'I wish I could help you, Mma,' said Mma Ramotswe. 'But I'm afraid I can't help everybody. I have not heard of this roof man. I'm sorry.'

The voice seemed to accept this and rang off, leaving Mma Ramotswe smiling. Really, people imagined that just because she was a detective she knew, or could find out, everything. It was an enviable reputation for a private detective to have, but it did mean that Mma Ramotswe was buttonholed in all sorts of unlikely circumstances and asked to come up with the solution to some often insoluble problem. If people had an issue to raise with a roofing man and had no other means of contacting him, then the answer seemed simple . . .

She picked up the telephone and redialled the number.

'I have thought of a possible solution,' she said. 'If this man fixes roofs, then why not drive around Gaborone and look for people fixing roofs. It is always very obvious whose roof is being fixed, because you will see a man standing on it. That is the way to find this man.'

The voice was silent for a moment. Then it let out a chuckle. 'What they say about you is obviously true, Mma,' said the voice. 'They say that you are a very clever lady – and you obviously are.'

It was a nice compliment to receive and Mma Ramotswe thought about it again that evening, when she prepared the evening meal for herself and Puso. It was strange there just being the two of them in the house, but it gave her an opportunity to talk more to Puso and find out what was going on at school. He was playing football, he said, and learning sums. He liked both of those but he did not like the hours they spent practising their handwriting. Having to do things like that when one was young, explained Mma Ramotswe, was necessary for when one was older.

'When you are big,' she said, 'and you write with very nice, neat handwriting, then you will thank that teacher who forced you to spend so much time practising. You will say, "He was a very good teacher and I am very grateful to him."'

'Never,' said Puso.

The next morning, when Mma Ramotswe came into the office after dropping Puso off at the school, she found Mma Makutsi already at her desk. On the way to school Puso had talked about football, and Mma Ramotswe had listened with only half an ear – if that. But at the end of the trip, as they approached the school gate, he had turned to her and said, 'What is that knocking sound, Mma? Is there somebody in the engine?'

'I think there is something loose,' said Mma Ramotswe. 'Maybe a nut and a bolt need to be tightened up. Mr J. L. B. Matekoni will do that in two minutes.'

'It is getting louder,' said Puso. 'Soon people will be shouting out, "Come in!" as you drive past.'

She had laughed the comment off, but it had worried her. If even Puso was beginning to notice that something was wrong with the tiny white van, then matters were indeed becoming serious. Sooner or later she would have to speak to Mr J. L. B. Matekoni about it, but she could not think about that

186

now, particularly since a development of an altogether more interesting stripe had occurred: there was something very different about Mma Makutsi.

It took Mma Ramotswe a moment or two to realise what had happened. As she entered the office, Mma Makutsi looked up from her desk and smiled at her, exchanging the normal, polite greeting. Mma Ramotswe returned the greeting and put the bag she was carrying down on her own desk. Then she stopped. It was Mma Makutsi, was it not? One takes so much for granted, in familiar surroundings at least, that one might quite easily enter a room and not take in the fact that an entirely unexpected person was there. Mma Makutsi's chair was occupied, but could it be somebody other than Mma Makutsi in it, some Mma Makutsi-looking person, but not the real Mma Makutsi; some relative or friend, perhaps, of the same general conformation?

She turned round slowly. 'Mma Makutsi?'

Again Mma Makutsi smiled broadly. 'Yes, Mma Ramotswe? How was Mma Potokwani yesterday? Still very bossy?'

It was well known that Mma Potokwani and Mma Makutsi, although civil enough to one another, did not see eye to eye on everything. In fact, they saw eye to eye on nothing. But now was not the time to go into that particular issue; now was the time to work out what it was that was so different about Mma Makutsi.

'Mma Makutsi,' said Mma Ramotswe. 'New glasses!'

Mma Makutsi reached up self-consciously and took off her glasses, examined them, polished them quickly on a small piece of cloth which she had taken out of a drawer, and then donned them again. 'Yes,' she said.

Mma Ramotswe was initially at a loss for words, her emotions mixed. Her assistant had several defining characteristics. One was the fact that she had achieved that ninety-seven per cent mark in the final examinations of the Botswana Secretarial College – an unequalled achievement in the annals of the college. Another was the fact that she came from Bobonong, which was in the middle of nowhere from the perspective of those who lived in Gaborone, if not of those who lived in Bobonong. And a further characteristic was that she wore extremely large, round glasses. All of these characteristics were quintessentially Mma Makutsi, to the extent that Mma Ramotswe felt that if the police were ever to need to issue a wanted description of Mma Makutsi – for some unimaginable secretarial offence – they would say, 'Wanted: woman from Bobonong, average height, ninety-seven per cent, large round glasses.' That would say everything and surely lead to her rapid detention. But now, without her round glasses, Mma Makutsi could walk with impunity through any police roadblock.

The new glasses were small. As Mma Ramotswe peered across the room at them she saw that whereas the previous glasses had reflected the surrounding light, this pair seemed to absorb it. And the frames were as different as could be imagined. The old frames had been made of a mock-tortoiseshell, predominantly brown; these were light blue, not far from the colour of one panel of Botswana's national flag, the blue which appeared on government buildings, at the gates of schools, or on the walls of more patriotically minded citizens.

'They are blue, Mma,' said Mma Ramotswe, struggling to find something to say. 'Botswana blue.'

'That is why I like them,' said Mma Makutsi. 'Or one of the reasons. The other reason is that they are very fashionable.'

Mma Ramotswe was quick to agree. She was uncertain what the current mode in glasses might be, but given that the requirements of fashion seemed to dictate that everything should become smaller, then these glasses were definitely following the trend. But the old glasses had character; they made Mma Makutsi what she was.

'I liked your old glasses, of course, Mma,' said Mma Ramotswe. 'They served you very well, I thought.'

Mma Makutsi gave a nonchalant wave of her hand. 'You have to move on, Mma. That is well known.'

Mma Ramotswe found herself agreeing. 'Of course,' she replied. 'People are always moving on. You can't stand still.' It was true, she supposed: people did move on and often used that expression to justify all sorts of questionable conduct. Husbands, in particular, had a tendency to move on when they reached a certain age and felt their youth slipping away from them. They moved on from their wives. And disloyal employees moved on, too, to better-paid jobs, even when they had been trained at the expense of their existing employer. There was, indeed, a lot of moving on.

And although she had glibly remarked that you could not stand still, was this actually true, or was it a hollow axiom, as false and misleading as any other trite saying? Why should one not stand still, if the position in which one found oneself standing was a satisfactory and comfortable one? She felt no need, no need at all, to move on from being Mma Ramotswe, of the No 1. Ladies' Detective Agency, wife of that great mechanic, Mr J. L. B. Matekoni. And Mr J. L. B. Matekoni himself had never moved on from anything, as far as she could ascertain, and would have been horrified were it to be suggested that he might do so. She imagined saying to him over the breakfast table, 'We must move on, Mr J. L. B. Matekoni. We really must.' He would look at his watch and say, 'Yes, my goodness, Mma Ramotswe, look at the time. I must get to the garage.'

And here was Mma Makutsi moving on from her old glasses and wearing this rather disconcertingly small, if highly fashionable, pair of blue ones. It was a very disorientating start to the day. She would get used to her assistant's new appearance, but for the time being she would ask Mma Makutsi to put on the kettle and make the first morning cup of tea. Or second, if one counted the cup of bush tea that Mma Ramotswe always enjoyed when she rose and walked around her garden while the sun floated gently above the horizon with its smiling; its benediction.

Mma Makutsi got up from her desk to put on the kettle. Mma Ramotswe saw – could not help spotting – that when Mma Makutsi spooned the tea into the teapot she missed, or partly missed, and some of the tea fell onto the floor. The ants would remove that; a tiny tea party for them, down in their miniature world. But Mma Ramotswe noticed it, and became thoughtful.

*

There were a few signs later on, but nothing that Mma Ramotswe could put her finger on. At mid-morning tea time, she watched closely, but Mma Makutsi delivered the tea with no difficulty and their attention, anyway, was focused on dealing with comments on the new glasses. Mr Polopetsi, of course, was polite, merely muttering, 'New spectacles, Mma,' but Charlie, hooting with laughter, said, 'Such small glasses, Mma! Does that make us all look very small? Are you sure you can see me, Mma? Look, here I am – over here. That tiny thing is me! And Mr Polopetsi, here, must be invisible – he's very small. Can you see him at all, Mma?'

Mma Ramotswe tended to ignore this sort of thing, and Mma Makutsi tried to do the same, but failed. She flashed an angry glance at Charlie and turned her back on him. Then a suitable retort occurred to her and she turned round to deliver it, but found herself face to face with Mr Polopetsi, who now became almost effusive in his remarks. 'Those are very nice glasses, Mma,' he said. 'Extremely pretty, in fact. There was a very small girl at the shops the other day wearing glasses just like those.'

Mma Makutsi acknowledged the compliment with a nod of her head, although she was not sure whether she should be pleased or annoyed with the last part of what Mr Polopetsi said. The rest of the tea break passed in a somewhat strained manner and Mma Ramotswe felt relieved when it was over and they could all get back to work. She had a few letters to dictate – and was Mma Makutsi hunched over her notebook more markedly than usual? She could not tell.

Then, half an hour or so later, Charlie came into the office. 'Letter for you, Mma Ramotswe,' he said. 'Somebody has just left it.'

People left notes for Mma Ramotswe, and she thought little of it. But when she took the envelope in her hands and began to slit open the flap, she felt a flush of foreboding. The letter was from that person; she could tell.

She read it carefully, aware of the fact that Mma Makutsi was watching her. *So, fat woman, you think you know everything! You and that assistant of yours, with her stupid glasses – you know nothing about what you don't know!*

Mma Makutsi was about to say something, but Mma Ramotswe anticipated her. 'Yes,' she said. 'It is another one.' And she thought: *which stupid glasses? The original stupid glasses, or the new stupid glasses?*

Mma Makutsi came over to take the letter. She peered at it, the paper close to her nose. *The glasses don't work!* Mma Ramotswe said to herself. But any satisfaction she might have experienced on having her earlier suspicions confirmed was eclipsed by the gravity of the moment.

Mma Makutsi walked over to the door that led into the garage. 'Charlie,' she shouted. 'Please come through here.'

Charlie appeared at the door, an adjustable wrench in his hand. 'I am very busy, Mma,' he said. 'What is it?'

'This letter, Charlie. You said that somebody left it. Who left it?'

Mma Ramotswe frowned. She knew the answer to Mma Makutsi's question; the letter would have been found on a surface somewhere in the garage, slipped there by Mr Polopetsi, so that it might be thought that somebody had dropped in unobserved. As a detective, even if only an assistant detective, Mma Makutsi should have realised that one could not assume that the letter had come from outside.

Charlie shrugged. 'Some woman,' he said. 'It was while we were dealing with that car under the tree – all of us. I came back to get something and I saw her coming out of the garage. I asked her what she wanted, but she just muttered something about making a mistake. Then she went off.'

Mma Ramotswe sat quite still. It was a woman. It was not Mr Polopetsi.

'Are you sure that she left it?' she asked. 'Are you sure it wasn't there before?'

Charlie seemed surprised that such interest was being taken in the details of what he thought was a very unimportant matter. What did it matter who left a letter? It would be perfectly obvious who had written it – letters bore signatures, after all. 'Yes, I am sure, Mma. It was on the petrol drum. I had been sitting on top of that before I went outside. There was no letter there. Then there was. It was that lady.'

'And you saw her face?' asked Mma Ramotswe.

'Yes,' said Charlie. 'She was a very pretty woman. Big bottom, too.'

'You think of nothing but bottoms,' snapped Mma Makutsi. 'You are like a little boy.'

'Oh yes,' said Charlie hotly. 'So there are lots of bottoms about. So that's my fault, is it?'

'You must not fight about . . . about unimportant things,' said Mma Ramotswe. 'It is not right.' She made a placatory gesture to Charlie. 'Now listen, Charlie, you didn't recognise this lady, did you? Had you seen her before?'

Charlie shook his head. 'No. Never.' He cast an angry glance at Mma Makutsi. 'Can I go now, Mma Ramotswe?'

'Of course you can, Charlie,' said Mma Ramotswe, adding, 'and thank you. Thank you for helping me to avoid making a big mistake.'

After Charlie had left, Mma Makutsi returned to sit down at her desk. She looked at the letter once more, and then shifted her gaze over to Mma Ramotswe. 'So, Mma Ramotswe,' she said. 'It was not Mr Polopetsi after all.'

Mma Ramotswe looked down at her hands – the hands of one who was capable, she realised, of the most appalling mis-judgement. 'I feel very bad, Mma,' she said. 'I feel very bad to have thought those things about him. It was very unfair.'

'Yes,' said Mma Makutsi. 'It was.'

Mma Ramotswe continued with her contemplation of her hands. She had made a mistake, but it was one which anybody might make in the face of the evidence that had been before her. And Mma Makutsi was not one to lecture her about making mistakes. Had she forgotten that bed left out in the rain? What about the new, unsuitable glasses?

She looked up. While she had been staring at her hands, Mma Makutsi, it seemed, had taken off her new glasses and slipped her old ones back on. Mma Ramotswe was momentar-ily taken aback by this, but recovered her composure. 'Yes,' she said to Mma Makutsi. 'We can all make mistakes, Mma. Even you.'

Nothing more was said. Mma Ramotswe's potentially disastrous mistake – fortunately not communicated to the entirely innocent Mr Polopetsi, whose embarrassment at forgetting he had a letter for her in his pocket she had taken for guilt – was cancelled out by Mma Makutsi's purchase of the unsuitable glasses. Both looked foolish. There need be no further mention of either matter, apart, perhaps, from one final question.

'Were they expensive, Mma?' asked Mma Ramotswe. 'Those glasses. Did they cost a lot?'

Mma Makutsi pursed her lips. They must have been very expensive, thought Mma Ramotswe.

Then Mma Makutsi said, 'I don't know, Mma.'

So Phuti Radiphuti bought them for her, thought Mma Ramotswe. That will lead to difficulties, as he will surely expect her to wear them.

Mma Makutsi realised that further explanation was necessary, and she now provided it. 'I found them, you see,' she said, her voice quiet, almost ashamed. 'I found them by the side of the road.'

It took Mma Ramotswe a little time to speak. 'You must—'

'Yes, I know,' interjected Mma Makutsi. 'I will hand them in. I was going to, I suppose. It's just that—'

'Good,' said Mma Ramotswe. 'So that's that.'

But it was not. Now came the thing that Mma Makutsi had not intended to tell Mma Ramotswe, but now it just tumbled out. 'I think I know who wears glasses like this,' she said, her voice barely above a whisper. 'Violet Sephotho!'

Mma Ramotswe gasped. 'Violet Sephotho! That horrid woman from the recruitment agency? The one who—'

'Yes,' said Mma Makutsi. 'That man-eater from the dancing class. The one who was rude about Phuti. The one who—'

'You have told me all about her,' said Mma Ramotswe. She hesitated. An idea was coming to her; just the germ of an idea. But she knew from experience that in these tiny, incipient ideas, these hunches, there often lay the answer to a major question.

'When did you find them?' she asked.

'A week ago,' said Mma Makutsi. 'Last Monday. I wasn't going to wear them, you see, and then . . .'

Mma Ramotswe held up a hand. She was not interested now in Mma Makutsi's struggles with her conscience. What she was interested in was finding out exactly where the glasses had been found. And the answer, when it came, confirmed what she had been thinking.

Chapter Fifteen

He Loved his Cattle.
He Loved his Country

Two days after Mr J. L. B. Matekoni had left for Johannes-burg with Motholeli, he telephoned Mma Ramotswe and told her at length about the trip and about their accommodation in a small hotel on the outskirts of the city. It was the second time that he had stayed in an hotel; for Motholeli it was the first. Both were excited.

'There is a very big bath in the bathroom,' Motholeli told Mma Ramotswe. 'And in the morning you can help yourself to as many eggs and as much bacon as you like. Mr J. L. B. Matekoni has been eating a lot.'

'Not that much,' she heard her husband saying in the background.

'And the doctors?' she asked.

'They are very kind,' said Motholeli.

Mma Ramotswe waited for something else to be said about the treatment, but neither Motholeli nor Mr J. L. B. Matekoni was forthcoming on the subject. 'They are doing a lot of things,' he said. 'I am not there, though, and so I cannot say what it is that they are doing.'

There was time enough to ponder this, and she did; rather too much, perhaps, as she found that anxiety over what was happening began to gnaw away at her. Now she started to reproach herself for not being firmer, for failing to veto a trip which she saw as pointless and even counter-productive. Motholeli had handled her disability with remarkable maturity and dignity; was it right, Mma Ramotswe wondered, that she should be encouraged to think that something could be done when it so obviously could not? Of course it would have been difficult to oppose the whole thing, for Mr J. L. B. Matekoni tended to hold on to an idea once he became attached to it. If she had refused to allow Motholeli to go to Johannesburg, then he could have ended up resenting her. So perhaps it was the right decision after all. On the other hand . . .

She had not asked how the trip and the treatment was to be paid for, and she might never have found out had Mma Makutsi not taken it upon herself during Mr J. L. B. Matekoni's absence to open the mail addressed to Tlokweng Road Speedy Motors. This was hardly voluminous – a few envelopes containing cheques for work done, a letter or two from suppliers of parts, advertisements for batteries – and a letter from the bank.

Mma Ramotswe could tell that there was something wrong when she saw her assistant frown. For a few moments she thought that perhaps the anonymous letter-writer had struck again, but then Mma Makutsi looked up and began to read. 'This is from the bank, Mma,' she said. 'This is what it says. "Dear Mr Matekoni, Further to your application for an un-secured loan, we regret to inform you that we shall, after all, require security for the sum for which you have applied. Our legal department will be in touch about setting up a bond over your garage premises to the extent of the sum applied for. This can be arranged within ten days of our receiving your instruc-tion . . ."' Mma Makutsi tailed off. 'He's going to mortgage the garage,' she said.

Mma Ramotswe got up from her desk and walked across the room to retrieve the letter. She read it through again, silently, and then returned it to its envelope. 'It's for Motholeli's treatment,' she said. 'That can be the only reason why he has applied for a loan.'

'Did he not tell you how much it would cost?' asked Mma Makutsi. 'That loan is for a lot of money, Mma. A lot. And if he fails to pay it back, then the bank takes the garage.'

Mma Ramotswe sighed. 'He is a kind man,' she said. 'He has always been a kind man.'

'Eee,' said Mma Makutsi. 'Eee, Mma.' It was really all that one could say in the face of such behaviour.

'But I can't let him do it,' said Mma Ramotswe. 'We cannot have a mortgage on this building. It is our main property.'

'And if we lost this building, then where would there be for the No. 1 Ladies' Detective Agency?' asked Mma Makutsi. 'We would be out on the street, along with the hawkers and the vegetable sellers. Can you imagine clients coming to an agency that was just a roadside stand?'

'They would not come,' said Mma Ramotswe. She imagined for a moment Mma Makutsi typing on a small, upturned wooden box, perhaps under a large blue umbrella to protect her from the sun, her ninety-seven per cent certificate from the Botswana Secretarial College leaning against the side of the box. No, it would not do.

'I shall have to get this money myself,' said Mma Ramotswe.

Mma Makutsi let out a low whistle. 'Have you got that much in your account, Mma? It is a lot of money.'

'No,' said Mma Ramotswe. 'I do not have that. Not in money.'

Mma Makutsi knew what Mma Ramotswe was going to say. 'Your cattle?'

There was silence. In Botswana, the sale or slaughter of one's cattle is the last resort; it is the last thing that anyone wishes to do. Cattle were the ultimate security, the property that stood before the very gates of indigence and kept them from opening. Once one had sold the cattle, there would be nothing left to sell.

Mma Ramotswe nodded her reply. 'I have a large herd,' she said. 'My daddy was very good with cattle. He left me

200

some very fine beasts, and they have multiplied. There are many of them now. I shall not have to sell all of them.'

'It is not a good thing to sell cattle,' said Mma Makutsi. 'Is there no other way, Mma?'

'I do not see one,' said Mma Ramotswe. 'I shall go out to the cattle post and choose the ones to sell.'

'This is a very sad day,' said Mma Makutsi.

'Yes,' said Mma Ramotswe. 'It is.' She would have liked to say that it was not, that there was a positive side to this; she was not one to concentrate on the bleak. But where was the positive side in having to dispose of those lovely animals, the legacy of her father, the grandchildren or great-grandchildren of the very cattle that had gathered round his house when in Mochudi he lay in his final illness; had gathered, she thought, to say goodbye to their owner?

But she would have to do it, and so she prepared the next day to go out to the cattle post, a journey of six hours on a very bumpy dirt road. She went in the tiny white van, and stopped halfway through the journey to eat a sandwich by the side of the road. It was mid-morning, and getting hotter. A hornbill watched her from the branch of a tree, casting his unnaturally large eye upon her. From another tree, some distance away, a lourie cried out with its distinctive call. She looked up at the sky. What was money? Nothing. A human conceit, so much smaller a thing than love, and friendship, and the pursuit, no matter how pointless, of hope. What did it matter that this money was being thrown away for no good reason? It mattered not at all, she decided.

And when, a few hours later, she stood with the man who looked after the cattle and identified those that she would sell, she did not think that it was the wrong thing to do, but picked them out bravely, without regret. That one, she said, and that one over there; that one is the calf of a cow my father called *the brave one*, that one came from far away, over that side, and was very strong; that one had a father who had only one horn. The cattle were rounded up, lowing, watching with their wide brown eyes, their heads moving to keep flies at bay; it was hot that afternoon and the trees themselves seemed to wilt; there was dust, kicked up by the cattle as they moved; there was the sound of bells tied round the necks of some of the herd. They are the ones who give music to the other cattle, her father had said of those ones.

Now that line came back to her, and she said it, under her breath. They are the ones who give music to the other cattle.

'What was that, Mma?' said the man. 'What did you say?'

Mma Ramotswe looked down at him; he was a short man, bow-legged, and his eyes were bright with intelligence. She smiled. 'It was something my daddy said. He was a man who knew a lot about cattle.'

The man inclined his head respectfully. 'I have heard that, Mma. I have heard people say that about him. They have said it.'

That Obed Ramotswe should be remembered, that people should still speak of him; that touched her. One did not have to be famous to be remembered in Botswana; there was room in history for all of us.

'He was a very good man,' she said. 'He loved his cattle. He loved his country.'

She had not intended to utter an epitaph, but that, she realised, was what she had done. And she thought: if your spirit is anywhere, then it is here, among your cattle, where you might hear what I have just said.

Chapter Sixteen

Mr Sekape Reveals some Peculiar Views

She had to decide. She could tell Mma Sebina first that she had found her brother, or she could speak to the brother, to this Mr Sekape, and reveal to him that he had a sister. The two possibilities raised quite distinct issues. Mma Sebina had asked her to find relatives for her; Mr Sekape had not. So while it would be no shock to Mma Sebina if Mma Ramotswe came up with a brother, that might not be the case with Mr Sekape. He would have got up that morning in the belief that he had no sister, and by the time he went to bed he would do so in the knowledge that he did have one. That would be a major change in his circumstances.

Mr Sekape Reveals some Peculiar Views

And yet that, surely, was what life was like. There would inevitably be certain days when things changed dramatically – days when we received bad news or good, which could dictate the shape of the rest of our lives. That had happened to her on that day, that fateful day, that Mr J. L. B. Matekoni had proposed to her, on the verandah of the house, as the sun went down. She had started that day without a fiancé and ended the day with one. And in Mma Makutsi's case there must have been a day, some time ago, when she had begun the day as an ordinary student of the Botswana Secretarial College and ended it as the college's most distinguished graduate in its entire history.

The news that one had a sister surely should be good news. It was possible that there were some people who did not want a sister, but she felt that there was no reason to assume that Mr Sekape would be one of these. Most people would be concerned that a newly discovered relative would make some sort of claim on them – a perfectly reasonable concern in a country where there was strong pressure to look after relatives. But Mma Sebina showed every sign of being quite well off and she would not be asking Mr Sekape for money. So there was no reason to hold back from telling him.

But what swayed her most was the fact that Mma Sebina might not be back until the following day, and Mma Ramotswe, quite simply, felt that she could not wait that long. The discovery was so thrilling that she wanted to tell somebody; no bearer of such momentous news could be expected to wait. So that decided that: she would go to the bank just before lunchtime and speak to Mr Sekape during his lunch hour. That would give him time to compose himself again for the start of the afternoon's business.

She parked the tiny white van near the museum; a shady place under a tree had just been vacated and she nosed into that, ignoring the knocking sound which continued to come from the engine. She would have to speak to Mr J. L. B. Matekoni about that when he came back, unless . . . she spoke to him first about the whining sound that his own truck seemed to make. If one had a mote in one's eye, then talking about the mote in another's could preclude discussion of one's own. She switched off the ignition and sat quite still as she contemplated the idea that had just occurred to her. If she managed to distract Mr J. L. B. Matekoni's attention from her van, then she could speak to Charlie about fixing it in his spare time. Charlie would not say anything about her having to get a new one, and, if he did, she could ignore his advice. And then if Mr J. L. B. Matekoni raised the subject, the tiny white van would be in good health again and there would be no awkward discussions about replacing it.

Cheered by the thought of this neat solution, Mma Ramotswe locked her van and crossed the road to the back of the Standard Bank. She looked at her watch anxiously; it was a few minutes before one and she hoped that Mr Sekape had not gone off for his lunch early. Even if he had, she would be able to find out where he had gone and seek him out there. But it would be easier to get him here, in the mall, where she could take him off to the President Hotel verandah a few yards away and make her disclosure.

She entered the bank. A security guard at the entrance looked her up and down and nodded to her.

'You have decided that I am not a bank robber,' said Mma Ramotswe.

The guard laughed. 'You are right, Mma,' he said. 'Bank robbers do not look at all like you. They're . . .' He tailed off, and looked to Mma Ramotswe for help.

Mma Ramotswe understood. 'You've never seen one, Rra? No? That's just as well, I think. We do not go in for bank robbers in Botswana.'

The guard looked relieved. 'I suppose I know what to do, which is nothing.'

Mma Ramotswe did not conceal her surprise, and the guard continued: 'I have been told that I must not try to disarm anybody who comes to rob the bank. I have to bear in mind the safety of the customers. That is the first thing I must do.'

Mma Ramotswe smiled. 'That is probably best, Rra. And anyway, here in Botswana if anybody came to rob the bank you'd probably know exactly who they were. You could simply threaten to tell their mothers. That would put a stop to any bank robbery.'

The guard clapped his hands together. 'Exactly, Mma! So my job is . . . is. . .' He could not bring himself to say unnecessary; nobody can be expected to admit that his job is unnecessary.

'Ceremonial,' said Mma Ramotswe. 'Your job is ceremonial.'

'That is what it is. Thank you, Mma.'

Mma Ramotswe acknowledged his thanks and moved on into the bank. Nearer pay day, at the end of the month, there would be long lines of people waiting for the tellers; now there were just a few customers at each of the windows. She looked around, made her way across the floor to a desk bearing a large *Enquiries* sign, and asked for Mr Sekape.

The woman behind the desk picked up a telephone and spoke a few words into the receiver. 'He will come down,' she said. 'He is upstairs, Mma. But you have caught him just before he goes out for lunch.'

Mma Ramotswe took a few steps backwards and waited. It is my job, she told herself; I am just doing my job. But the significance of what she was about to tell Mr Sekape made her heart beat faster, her mouth feel dry.

She told him that she had some news for him, that it was not bad news, but that she would need to talk to him outside. Could he join her out in the square? As they walked, they could talk. He was not to be alarmed; it was something that she thought he would be happy to hear.

He was not alarmed, nor even surprised by her request. In a country where news was often conveyed by messenger, it was not unusual for a stranger to announce that there was something they needed to discuss. There were a hundred things that might be talked about on such an occasion: difficulties with marriage negotiations, problems over the custody or education of a child, matters relating to cattle; it could be anything.

'It's getting hotter,' said Mr Sekape as they moved out from the shade of the bank building. 'There will be more rain soon, I think.'

'I hope so,' said Mma Ramotswe. 'I was on the Lobatse Road the other day and there was a lot of green. And the dam too – I have read in the newspapers that the level is getting higher.'

'That is all very good,' said Mr Sekape. 'This is all very good news.'

But it is not this news that you have brought me, Mma, he thought. You have not come to talk about the rains.

She glanced at him sideways, taking in the neat appearance, the black trousers with the thin leather belt, the polished shoes. He was exactly as she had imagined he would be, a mid-level employee of the bank, doing well, heading for promotion to branch manager at some point. Such lives were quietly and correctly led to the very edge of the grave; lives of caution and respectability, with few high points and moments of excitement. She allowed her glance to move to his left hand: no ring. That was not conclusive, of course, but it was surprising; she would have expected a ring.

They walked slowly up the centre of the square that opened up in front of the President Hotel. Traders had set out their wares on the large concrete flagstones that covered the square, the goods ranged out carefully on sheets of plastic or sacking: roughly made sandals, wooden carvings, lines of glistening sunglasses. They passed a dealer in traditional medicines who had created small piles of herbs, roots, barks, crushed leaves. Mma Ramotswe looked down and saw a root that she recognised, that she had been given to chew as a girl, which worked, she thought, for something that she had forgotten about – a sore stomach, perhaps. She leaned down and asked the woman selling the herbs whether that was for the stomach and the woman nodded. 'You have a pain, Mma? In your stomach?'

'I have no pain, Mma. But I know that is a good thing, that one. It is very good.'

Mr Sekape said nothing. He wanted to hear what she had to say to him; he was not interested in old roots.

Mma Ramotswe straightened up. 'You were adopted, Rra,' she said. 'Mma Potokwani has told me.'

Mr Sekape stopped, and stiffened. 'That is true, Mma. I was very small. I was looked after by a lady who lived right here in Gaborone. She was a teacher at the secondary school. She became my mother.'

'And her husband?'

He shook his head. 'He was late by the time she took me. He worked for the government, in the Ministry of Education. She had a small pension from them, but her own job was a good one. She gave me everything.'

They started to walk again. His initial stiffness of manner when she had first raised the matter of his adoption had eased, and he began to talk more freely. 'She is late now. Three years ago. I still miss her, because I carried on living in her house right up to the end. Now I have that house to myself.'

Mma Ramotswe made a sympathetic sound, something between *yes* and *I see*. 'You must miss her.' And she thought of her own father, whom she missed.

And that was what she was thinking – of Obed Ramotswe and of her father's cousin, who had, all those years ago, given her a root to chew for a sore stomach – when Mr Sekape stopped, and touched her lightly on the arm, and asked, 'What is it, Mma? What have you come to tell me?'

And now that the moment had come, she replied, without thinking of how she might put it, 'I have come to tell you that you have a sister, Rra. I do not think that you know about her, but you have a sister.'

She heard him catch his breath. She saw his hand go to his face, to somewhere near his mouth, and then drop again.

'Yes, Rra. This lady, your sister, has come to me and asked me to find her family. And I have found you.'

At first he said nothing. He turned his face away, to look in the direction of the government buildings at the other end of the square, and she thought, this is not welcome news for him, but then, when he turned back to face her, there was no mistaking the emotion within him. His voice cracked as he spoke; he stopped to compose himself. 'You have found me a sister, Mma? You have found her?'

'I have, Rra. I can take you to her. I can take you to her . . .' She shrugged. 'Tomorrow, maybe. Or the day after. I can do that.'

He was looking down at the ground. Behind him, two women were walking slowly across the square, carrying bags stuffed with purchases. One of the women looked up, and Mma Ramotswe recognised her; a friend of Sister Banjule at the Anglican hospice, who had nursed Mma Makutsi's brother

211

in his final days; by these bonds of friendship are we linked, one to another.

'*Dumela, Mma Ramotswe.*'

'*Dumela, Mma.*' Mma Ramotswe did not know the other woman's name, but it did not matter; the two passed on and she was left with Mr Sekape, who looked up.

'No, Mma,' he said. 'Please take me today. Please take me now. I cannot wait.' He looked about him. 'I must buy her a present. I must . . .'

He seemed flustered, and Mma Ramotswe took his hand. 'There will be plenty of time for that, Rra. A whole lifetime, don't you think?'

Mma Ramotswe would have liked to have had more time to arrange the meeting with Mma Sebina, but Mr Sekape was insistent. They could not wait, he said, because anything could happen; there could be a road accident, there could be a storm, and the meeting might never take place; none of us, he said, can be completely sure of seeing the next day. And what a waste of her hard work it would be, he said, if this sister were to be snatched away from him just when he had discovered her. That, thought Mma Ramotswe, was perhaps being some-what pessimistic; neither of them was aged, neither of them seemed afflicted by ill health; one day, surely, would not matter. But she did not voice these objections. She might have hoped to give Mma Sebina more warning, to give her time to get used to the existence of a brother, but she could not say no to Mr Sekape in his almost boyish enthusiasm, because if she did, it crossed her mind, the disaster that he feared might just occur. There might be an accident, and then . . .

It was because he was a man, she thought, that he could not wait; men were not very good about keeping presents, but wanted to open them immediately. Women could wait, could enjoy the slow build-up of excitement. We are different, she thought; we are definitely different. Whatever people said about everybody being the same, it simply was not true. There were profound and obvious differences between men and women and the way in which they viewed the world. These existed; they simply did.

Mr Sekape returned to the bank and excused himself for the afternoon. Then, travelling together in the tiny white van, they made their way back to the agency.

'My assistant will look after you while I go to look for your sister,' said Mma Ramotswe. 'I hope that I can find her quickly and bring her to you.'

'You will find her quickly,' said Mr Sekape. 'I have a feeling that you will find her very quickly.'

Mma Ramotswe took her eyes off the road briefly to look at him. 'I hope so,' she said. He was like a schoolboy, she thought; as impetuous as a schoolboy. And what else? She had ascertained in their earlier conversation that there was no wife, which was unusual. He was obviously not hard up, and he had a house. Why, then, no wife? She knew that it was often hard for women, with the shortage of men, but if a man had a bit of money and a house, then he could take his pick of suitable women, who would be only too pleased to marry him.

She remembered her policy of asking. Time and time again she had proved the proposition that if one wanted the answer to anything, then one should simply ask. It was simple, and she wondered whether the police were sufficiently aware of the attractions of such an approach. If they were investigating a crime they should simply stop and ask, 'Who did this?' and they would surely be given the answer – perhaps even from the criminal himself, who might just stand up and say, 'I did it, Rra.' Or perhaps not.

'Did you never want to get married, Rra?' she asked, as she negotiated their way round the traffic circle near the football stadium.

Mr Sekape looked out of the window. For a few moments she thought that he was not going to answer, but then, transferring his gaze to his hands, folded upon his lap, he said, 'No. Never. Not once, Mma. Never.'

It was a clear enough answer, thought Mma Ramotswe. Some answers were evasive and ambiguous; this was not.

Coming out of the traffic circle, she brought the van back onto a straight course. There was that noise again, that knocking; it seemed to get louder when she pressed her foot on the accelerator pedal, and retreated when she took it off.

'Why not, Rra?'

Unlike her earlier question, which had been thought about before being asked, this question slipped out. It was not the sort of question that she would normally ask; she would not have liked anybody to ask her, before she became engaged to Mr J. L. B. Matekoni, why she was not married. And after their engagement, she certainly resented being asked – as she sometimes was – why the engagement was lasting so long and no firm date had been set for the wedding.

Mr Sekape continued to study his hands. 'It's because I do not like women,' he said. 'That is why. I do not like them. Sorry, Mma, but you asked me. So now I am telling you. They are always talking, talking, talking. Asking you this thing. Asking you that. That is why I do not like them.'

The tiny white van swerved, very slightly, but still swerved, as Mma Ramotswe tightened her grip on the wheel. She wanted to say, but did not, 'I think I should tell you, Rra – this sister I've found for you – she's a woman. You do know that, don't you?'

Chapter Seventeen

An Unusual Chase in an Unusual Place

Two days passed – two days in which more rain fell, great cloudbursts of rain, drenching the length and breadth of Botswana. People held their breath in gratitude, hardly daring to speak of the deluge lest it should suddenly stop and the dryness return. The rivers, for long months little more than dusty beds of rust-coloured sand, appeared again, filled to overflowing in some cases, twisting snakes of mud-brown water moving across the plains. Here and there low bridges were overwhelmed by the floods and were covered with fast-moving water, cutting off villages and settlements from the larger roads; but nobody complained. The bush, a desiccated brown before the storms, turned green overnight, as the shoots of dormant plants thrust their way through the soil. Flowers followed, tiny yellow flowers, spreading like a dusting of gold across the land. Ground vines sent out tendrils; melons would grow in abundance later on, as an offering, an expiation for the barrenness of the dry months that had gone before.

For Mma Ramotswe, those two days of rain were days of waiting. There was work enough for her to attend to – several matters that for some time she had been meaning to finish off were calling for attention – and Mma Makutsi, too, had things to do. She had been handling the case of the tenant who was not who he claimed to be, and there was a report to be written on that. She and Phuti had followed the man staying in the house, driving behind him discreetly in Phuti's white car with the red stripe down the side. That had gone smoothly enough and they had seen the tenant go into the office of a supplier of diesel generators, exactly where the informing neighbour had said that he worked. But was he the Mr Moganana who was named in the lease, or was he his brother-in-law, who had no right to be staying in the house? That had been solved by Phuti, who had gone into the office and asked to speak to Mr Moganana. He had expected to be told that no such person worked there; instead the man they had followed had appeared. Phuti, unprepared for this, had simply asked him whether he was the man who had leased the house in question.

'Of course I am, Rra,' Mr Moganana replied. 'And a real dump it is too. Are you from the landlord?'

'In a way,' said Phuti.

217

'Well, you can tell her that I am fed up with her never doing anything about that bathroom.'

'Is there something wrong, Rra?'

'There certainly is. If it weren't for the fact that I've signed that lease I would leave tomorrow.'

And that had solved that. The client would be told that if she wanted the house back, all she had to do was to cancel the lease; both sides would be pleased. It was one of those cases where both sides appeared to win, and everybody ended up happy.

For his part, Phuti enjoyed the experience, and dropped broad hints that he was at the agency's disposal at any time they needed his services. Mma Makutsi had smiled, and promised to pass the message on to Mma Ramotswe. And then, in the glow of warmth over a job well done, she had confessed to him about the bed.

'It is the second bed,' she said. 'The one you have taken from the garage and put into storage is the second bed. I ruined the first. It was all my fault.'

He had listened sympathetically, and taken her hand at the end of the story. 'I thought that there was something odd about it,' he said. 'But I didn't like to ask. This one has a different pattern on the headboard. I noticed that straight away. And . . .'

She caught her breath. What would he think of her for not having told him before? Perhaps she should tell him that she had simply forgotten to do so, but that would be another lie, and she was ashamed enough of the first one.

'I knew that you did it so that I should not be upset,' said Phuti. 'You were very kind.'

Mma Makutsi said nothing.

'You are so kind to me,' said Phuti. 'I am a very fortunate man.'

The writing of the report on their case kept Mma Makutsi busy for a time, but once that was done she seemed to pick up the unease which was affecting her employer and she took it upon herself to engage in a restless sorting through of old files and refiling them according to a new system that she was in the process of developing. Both of them drank too much tea; the act of putting on the kettle and making the tea was at least a ritual which could divert them for twenty minutes or so, and if one did it often enough a morning or an afternoon would slip by quickly enough.

At least Mma Ramotswe knew the cause, or rather the causes, of her unease. Mr J. L. B. Matekoni and Motholeli were due back in two days' time, and she was anxious about their return. But there was more than that. She had made the occasional mistake in her professional life, she was not perfect, but the mistake that she felt she had made in introducing Mma Sebina to Mr Sekape was, she thought, one of the more serious ones. I should have been more careful, she told herself; I should have thought about it. I should have spoken to them both separately before I introduced them. I should have done everything differently. Such thoughts now played on her mind, and she considered each one of them in turn, and then went back to the first and started again.

For something very bad had happened; something that now placed her, she felt, in an impossible position. This new development was not entirely her fault; if anybody should be blamed it was Mma Potokwani, but the redoubtable matron of the orphan farm was showing herself to be quite cavalier in her attitude to what she had done; there had been no apology from that quarter. And now Mma Ramotswe would have to do something about it – there was no doubt in her mind about that – but she could not bring herself to face the prospect. Like an animal in the lights of an oncoming car, she found herself incapable of moving.

She turned to Mma Makutsi for help. Her assistant was sympathetic, immediately launching into spirited criticism of Mma Potokwani, whom she had always regarded as excessively pushy and – 'Did I not tell you, Mma Ramotswe?' – now downright irresponsible. But Mma Makutsi did not volunteer to do for Mma Ramotswe the thing that she was dreading; Mma Ramotswe would have to do that herself.

'You'll have to go and see her,' said Mma Makutsi. 'I'm sorry, Mma, but there's no other way. You'll have to go and see Mma Sebina and tell her.'

Mma Ramotswe groaned inwardly. 'I know, Mma. You're quite right. I cannot run away from this.'

'Of course it's all Mma Potokwani's fault, Mma,' Mma Makutsi went on, shaking her head in disbelief. 'You would think, wouldn't you, Mma Ramotswe, that when it came to something as important as that she would bother to check her facts. But did she? She did not, Mma! She said to you, just like

220

that, "Oh yes, I remember those children. I remember that there were two – a brother and a sister." And then she phones up and says, "Oh, Mma Ramotswe, there has been a mistake. That man, that Mr Sekape who works at the Standard Bank, he was not the brother of the girl who went to Otse. The brother of that girl died when she was still quite young. I am sorry, Mma, but that means she has no brother." How could she do that, Mma? How could she be so stupid?'

Mma Makutsi stared at Mma Ramotswe in triumph: there could be no defence for Mma Potokwani, none at all. And as she thought this, she glanced down at her shoes, her green shoes with the sky-blue linings, and it seemed to her that even her shoes, contrary as they were at times, agreed with her. *Quite right, Boss! Mma Potokwani's shoes are pretty stupid too! Stupid lady, stupid shoes!*

'Oh, I know it's a silly mistake,' said Mma Ramotswe. 'But it must be easy enough to make, with all those children going through her hands. I don't know how she remembers all their names.'

'She doesn't,' said Mma Makutsi simply. 'She gets them wrong. As we have seen.'

Mma Ramotswe wanted to defend her old friend against such attack, but could not; she felt too miserable for that. She knew, too, that from whatever angle she considered the matter, the answer would be the same: she would have to go to Mma Sebina and announce that she had not found her brother after all. And then she would have to tell Mr Sekape too that there had been a misunderstanding and he was, once again, alone.

When she first heard about Mma Potokwani's mistake, her initial thought was that it might not be a bad thing after all. The meeting that she had set up between Mma Sebina and Mr Sekape had not been the success she had envisaged, and at first she wondered whether Mma Sebina, having found a brother, would prove to be quite happy to lose him again. After all, when she had eventually located Mma Sebina and brought her to the office to meet Mr Sekape, the encounter between the two long-lost siblings had been far from the emotionally charged reunion Mma Ramotswe had expected. Mr Sekape had stood up, barely looking at his new-found sister, and had extended his hand for a formal handshake. For her part, Mma Sebina had been largely silent, replying to his questions in a voice which both Mma Ramotswe and Mr Sekape himself had had to struggle to hear. There had been no effusive expressions of sentiment; no exchanges of embraces; just rather stiff social formalities. Where did you go to school, Mma? Did you ever meet anybody who knew our mother? Do you think that we might have some uncles on our father's side? These were the questions which formed the conversation between the two.

And at the back of Mma Ramotswe's mind, as she listened to this, was the thought of what Mr Sekape had said earlier on in the van. Mma Ramotswe understood that there were some men who did not like women, just as there were some women who did not like men. But she had never encountered somebody who had spelled that out so clearly; and even if one were to give Mr Sekape some credit for honesty, all that credit would rapidly be offset by the discredit he would get for writing off half of humanity in such firm and unfriendly terms. If he were my brother, thought Mma Ramotswe, I would settle that issue right at the beginning.

The meeting between the two of them had not lasted long. After about half an hour or so, silence had set in, and Mma Sebina had given Mma Ramotswe a glance of the sort that one woman can give another which signals that help is required. Mma Ramotswe had then said something about how time was marching on and that if Mr Sekape did not mind she would now run him back to the bank in her van. This offer had been accepted, and then the two had exchanged telephone numbers.

'I shall telephone you tonight,' said Mr Sekape.

And Mma Sebina had replied, 'I shall be there, Rra. I shall answer.'

No, it had been a stiff meeting, a disappointment, and Mma Ramotswe had decided that she would not be surprised if the relationship fizzled out altogether. There were brothers and sisters, after all, who saw one another infrequently and did not seem to mind if they only met at family weddings and funerals. Perhaps this is how it would be for them.

But it was not. This gloomy prognosis had to be revised the following day when Mma Sebina telephoned Mma Ramotswe and told her that the two of them had met again on the very evening of their first encounter.

'He came to my house, Mma,' she said, 'and I made him a very good meal. He said that he had not had anybody to cook for him since his mother became late. He was very happy.'

'I am glad about that,' said Mma Ramotswe. So at least Mr Sekape accepted that women could have some uses, even if he professed to have such a low opinion of them. Mind you, she thought, all men who dislike women leave their dislike at the kitchen door.

'Yes,' enthused Mma Sebina. 'And we had a very good time. He told me some very funny stories about the bank. He has a good sense of humour. I have often wondered if people who work in banks laugh much. Now I know they do.'

Mma Ramotswe was too surprised to say anything to this. Perhaps Mr Sekape's self-confessed hostility to women did not extend to sisters; perhaps he had discovered that his dislike was not as intense as he had imagined it to be. Or perhaps she had misunderstood him altogether, and his surprising remark had not been intended to be taken seriously. Whatever the explanation was, it was a welcome development: Mma Ramotswe did not like to disappoint clients and it seemed that Mma Sebina was more than happy with the outcome of the encounter.

And that, of course, made her task of breaking the present news all the more difficult. But she had to do it, and had at last plucked up sufficient courage to go and speak to Mma Sebina.

'I shall go right now,' she said to Mma Makutsi. 'I have put the matter off for long enough. I shall go, Mma—'

And that is the moment at which Charlie burst in. He did not knock, as even he normally did; he burst in.

'I've seen her,' he announced breathlessly. 'I've just seen her.'

Mma Makutsi sniffed in an irritated way. 'Seen who?' she snapped. 'And have you forgotten how to knock, Charlie?'

Charlie ignored her and addressed his next remark to Mma Ramotswe. 'That woman who brought the letter,' he said. 'I have just seen her go into the supermarket. You seemed so interested in her that I rushed back to tell you. But since Mma Makutsi seems to be more concerned about knocking and such things perhaps I should not have bothered.'

Mma Ramotswe stood up. 'Charlie,' she said, 'we must go there now. You. Me. Mma Makutsi. Straight away.'

There was not enough room for all three of them in the tiny white van, and so Charlie crouched in the back, clinging on to the side, while Mma Ramotswe and Mma Makutsi occupied the driver's and passenger's seat respectively. The van was making the suspicious knocking noise again, but that did not stop Mma Ramotswe from pressing the accelerator pedal flat to the floor. Even so, with the engine doing its utmost, there was no question of reaching such momentum as would break the speed limit, and Mma Ramotswe found herself glancing anxiously at her watch as they made their way along the Tlokweng Road in the direction of the Pick and Pay supermarket.

Fortunately the traffic, such as it was, was going in the opposite direction, streaming away from town, and there was little to hold them up. When they reached the lights at the southern edge of the village, the tiny white van was brought to a halt dutifully at the line.

'It's a pity the lights are red,' said Mma Makutsi. 'When you

225

see detectives in films they do not let these things hold them up.'

Mma Ramotswe glanced from left to right. Everything was clear; there were no vehicles approaching.

'But it's the law, Mma Makutsi,' she said. 'You cannot have people deciding whether or not they will stop at lights. That is not the way we do things in Botswana – yet.'

'I was not saying that you should jump the lights, Mma,' said Mma Makutsi, somewhat huffily. 'I do not jump the lights myself.'

'But you don't drive,' observed Mma Ramotswe. 'You can't jump lights if you don't drive.'

'When I am with Phuti,' said Mma Makutsi. 'What I meant was that Phuti and I don't jump lights. We always stop when the lights are red. Even when they are orange, we stop.'

Mma Ramotswe looked in both directions again. There was still nothing coming.

'Of course, if it's an emergency,' she said hesitantly. 'If one is heading somewhere to solve a crime, for example. Or taking a pregnant lady to the hospital. Then I think that it's all right to go against the lights. As long as you've looked, of course.'

Mma Makutsi looked up the road. 'Do you think that this is an emergency, Mma?'

'Well, writing threatening letters is a crime, I think,' said Mma Ramotswe. But she was not completely sure of that. She had a copy of the Botswana Penal Code in the office, which she occasionally waved at any client who might suggest doing something illegal – such as listening to the telephone calls of another – but was there anything in the code about threatening letters? There should be, she felt, but then there were many things that should be in the Botswana Penal Code but were not, because of some oversight on the part of the compilers – failing to support an indigent parent, for example, or conducting a loud telephone conversation on the verandah of the President Hotel when other people were trying to drink their tea in peace.

The lights changed, and they moved forward. Within a few moments they were in the parking area and she nosed the tiny white van into the nearest vacant space, switched off the ignition, and began to half run towards the supermarket entrance, accompanied by Charlie and Mma Makutsi.

'We must get a trolley,' said Mma Makutsi, as they entered. 'We must be careful to look like normal shoppers. Then we shall be able to see this person and observe her.'

'And then?' asked Charlie. 'Should I detain her?'

Mma Makutsi scoffed. 'You cannot detain people, Charlie. You are not a policeman! No, what we shall do is follow her and find out who she is. That's what we should do, isn't it, Mma Ramotswe?'

Mma Ramotswe had not thought that far. 'I think so,' she said. 'We will observe, I think.'

They moved towards the vegetable section. Charlie's offer to push the trolley had been turned down by Mma Ramotswe, who thought it better for her to remain in control. Mma Makutsi walked beside her, one hand on the trolley bar.

'Do you mind if I pick up a few things as we go along?'

227

asked Mma Makutsi. 'I was going to have to come shopping later on, anyway. So I may as well get something for Phuti's dinner while I'm about it.'

Mma Ramotswe agreed that this was a good idea. 'But don't spend too much time choosing,' she said. 'She could almost have finished her shopping by now, and so we had better get down towards the end of the store as soon as possible.'

The supermarket was not busy, although there were short lines of people at the bakery and meat sections. They avoided these, and walked instead down the curry and pasta lanes. Mma Makutsi reached for a jar of peri-peri sauce and put it into the tray.

'Phuti likes peri-peri chicken,' she explained. 'He has a taste for hot things.'

'I can't stand it,' said Charlie. 'Why spoil good food by making it so hot that it burns your mouth? What's so good about having a burnt mouth, Mma Makutsi?'

'It doesn't really burn your mouth,' Mma Makutsi replied. 'It just tastes like that.'

'Same thing,' said Charlie.

Mma Ramotswe was eager to return to the business in hand. 'Let's not argue about such matters,' she said. 'Everybody likes different things. We are not all made the same way.'

They were approaching the tea section, and Mma Ramotswe began to slow down, her attention drawn to a display of brightly coloured boxes of tea. 'Now that looks very nice,' she said. 'Perhaps—'

She did not finish. Charlie had seen something; now he abruptly reached out and clapped his hand over hers on the trolley bar. 'There she is, Mma! There. Look.'

They stood quite still. At the end of the lane, on the point of turning the corner, was a woman in a shiny green dress, pushing a trolley laden with foodstuffs.

It was Mma Makutsi who broke the silence. 'Violet!' she exclaimed. 'Violet Sephotho!'

Mma Makutsi's voice carried, at least as far as Violet, who spun round to find out who it was who had called her name. For a moment she appeared confused, but then, turning sharply on her heel, she changed the direction of her shopping trolley and began to push it towards the household products section. Mma Ramotswe lost no time. Leaning into the trolley, she began to pursue Violet, the trolley wheels clattering noisily as they picked up speed.

After a few seconds, Violet half turned to glance behind her. Seeing herself pursued by Mma Ramotswe's advancing trolley, she spun her own trolley round the approaching corner. For a short while she was out of sight of her pursuers, but Mma Ramotswe was now assisted in the pushing of the trolley by Mma Makutsi and Charlie and they began rapidly to close the distance between them.

'Violet Sephotho!' called out Mma Makutsi. 'You stop right now! You stop! In the name of . . .' In the name of what? she thought. And it came to her, even if she did not utter the words: *In the name of the Botswana Secretarial College.* Violet Sephotho had been her contemporary there, the leader of the glamorous girls, the seditious, lazy one who sat at the back of the classroom and read magazines. Mma Makutsi had not forgotten how it was Violet who had pretended to snore during a lecture on double-entry bookkeeping by a very important visitor, the secretary of the Botswana Association of Certified Accountants. Neither had Mma Makutsi forgotten the stream of eligible boyfriends paraded so shamelessly on Violet's arm; nor the moment when she had announced that she had landed the best-paid job of that year's graduates in spite of her appallingly bad examination results. And now she was revealed as the author of those unpleasant letters. But why, she wondered, would she have done that?

Violet showed no sign of stopping, but then, turning a corner past an elaborate display of stacked boxes of soap powder, she slipped. She righted herself quickly, but it was enough to send her trolley into the pile of boxes, which tumbled about her in a cloud of white powder. More from surprise than from anything else, she stood where she was, allowing Mma Ramotswe and Mma Makutsi to catch up with her.

'We need to talk to you, Mma,' said Mma Ramotswe.

'About those letters,' interjected Mma Makutsi. 'It was you, wasn't it?'

'I don't know what you're talking about,' said Violet.

Mma Makutsi's eyes were wide. 'You don't? Those letters addressed to Mma Ramotswe. The ones that made those remarks about us. Those ones. You don't know anything about them?'

Violet dusted soap powder off her dress. 'No, I don't. I

have no idea what you're talking about, Grace Makutsi. I really don't.'

'Then why did you run away from us, Mma?' asked Mma Ramotswe. She spoke calmly, and there was about her demeanour none of the outrage that had so obviously seized Mma Makutsi.

Violet hesitated. 'Was I running away, Mma? What made you think I was running away?'

'But you were!' shouted Mma Makutsi.

'You saw us, and you ran away,' said Mma Ramotswe. 'It did look a bit like that, Mma.'

For a few moments Violet said nothing. Then she laughed. 'Oh, I see how you thought that. There's a simple explanation, you know – even if it will be a bit hard for some of you to get into her head.' At this, she looked at Mma Makutsi, before continuing, 'You see, I thought you were somebody else altogether. I thought that you were somebody who . . . well, I owe a bit of money to. I'm going to pay them back next month, but I didn't want them to make a scene here, in public. So I decided to get away from them. Simple, you see.'

Mma Ramotswe studied Violet as she spoke. It was hard to judge, she thought. Most liars were transparent, but the really hardened ones, the ones who were cold inside, who felt nothing, could lie very convincingly precisely because they felt no guilt. Everything that she had heard about Violet suggested that she was a person of that sort, and so all this might be lies – or it could be truth; she simply could not tell. And yet there still were questions she could ask.

231

'Tell me, Mma,' she asked gently, 'why did you think that we were those other people? Do we look like them? Is one of them a traditionally built person? And one a young man like this one here? Or one like Mma Makutsi?'

Violet frowned, as if trying to make sense of the question. Then her answer came. 'I cannot see very well in the distance at the moment,' she said. 'I have lost my glasses, you see.'

The look that Mma Makutsi exchanged with Mma Ramotswe was so obvious, so triumphant, that even Violet noticed it.

'So?' said Violet. 'So what's so odd about that?'

'Blue frames?' asked Mma Makutsi, leaning forward towards Violet as she spoke. 'Small glasses with blue frames?'

'No, not those ones,' said Violet. 'I have those with me here, not that it's any of your business, Grace Makutsi. My other glasses. The ones I use for long distance.'

And with that, she took a small pair of blue glasses out of the pocket of her dress, polished them ostentatiously, and then put them away.

Chapter Eighteen

There are Many Miracles

'It was her,' said Mma Makutsi, as she filled Mma Ramotswe's cup with tea and placed it on her desk, with rather more force, perhaps, than normally. 'Of course it was her! Charlie was sure it was the same woman who had dropped off the letter. You heard him, Mma.'

Mma Ramotswe lifted the cup to her lips and looked down into the dark red-brown liquid. It seemed troubled; when Mma Makutsi made tea in a bad mood, the tea reflected this. She sighed. She did not like to quote Clovis Andersen too often, but this, surely, was an occasion when the words of *The Principles of Private Detection* were particularly apposite.

'Clovis Andersen,' Mma Ramotswe began, 'says that you should never rely entirely on an identification. I remember his exact words, Mma Makutsi. *The human memory plays all sorts of tricks. You may think that you remember correctly, but you might not. Remember that people are very similar to one another – we all have arms and legs and noses, and these can look very, very alike.* That's what he says, Mma.'

Mma Makutsi listened in silence. She was not one to argue with Clovis Andersen, but in this case, even if Charlie's identification were to be discounted, Violet Sephotho was such an obvious suspect. The only matter to be sorted out was motive, and that, when one started to think about it, was clear enough. Envy. The last time the paths of the two women had crossed, Violet had shown herself to be envious of Phuti. She disparaged him, of course, and made fun of his awkwardness and his speech impediment, but the fact remained: Phuti was well off. Violet would have loved to have married a rich man, but presumably had failed. For her to see Mma Makutsi, whom she despised, with a rich fiancé on her arm must have been more than she could bear. And the hostile references to Mma Ramotswe? A smokescreen intended to conceal the real target: Mma Makutsi, fiancée of the proprietor of the Double Comfort Furniture Shop – and of a very large herd of cattle.

Mma Makutsi was so sure that Violet was the author of the letters that it frustrated her that Mma Ramotswe should not grasp this point. But in this she was mistaken; Mma Ramotswe did, in fact, think that it was Violet, it was just that she was

reluctant to say that it had been *established* that she was the cul-
prit. This point was now explained to Mma Makutsi.

'I agree, you know,' said Mma Ramotswe. 'It was probably
Violet Sephotho. The glasses were nothing to do with the case.
And the reason why I believe that Charlie really was correct is
this: Charlie looks at women very carefully. He studies them –
we have all seen that. And he said something very significant,
Mma. He said that when he saw her pushing the trolley in the
supermarket – he saw her from behind, remember – he was
more convinced than ever. He said that . . . well, it's a bit indelicate, Mma, but I have to say it. He said that it was the same
bottom.'

Mma Ramotswe's embarrassment appeased Mma Makutsi,
who let out a whoop of laughter. 'That boy! That is all he ever
thinks of. But this time, he was right. Good for Charlie!'

It was a tiny compliment – *good for Charlie* – the sort of
thing that might be said without really meaning anything, but
it was the first time Mma Ramotswe had heard Mma Makutsi
say something positive about the apprentice, and she was
struck by it. Something had happened; some sandbank of ani-
mosity had shifted, even if slightly.

Mma Makutsi brought her back to the matter in hand. 'But
what do we do, Mma Ramotswe?'

'We write to Violet,' she said. 'We send a letter, which I shall
dictate after I have finished my tea.'

Mma Makutsi showed her satisfaction at this. 'Oh, that is a
very good idea, Mma. We can inform her that we have handed
the letters over to the police. We can also say that we have

consulted our lawyers and that they are preparing a case against her. And we can tell her that we are not surprised to hear that the letters were written by such a silly, cowardly person, who was a disgrace to the Botswana Secretarial College – a complete disgrace.'

Mma Ramotswe shook her head. 'No, Mma. I don't think we shall do that. Thank you, but no.' She picked up her cup and drained the last of the tea from it. I'm going to need all the support of this tea, she thought, as after this letter I am going to have to go and see Mma Sebina.

Mma Makutsi readied her notebook. 'I am ready, Mma.'

Mma Ramotswe cleared her thoat. 'Dear Violet,' she began. 'We met in the supermarket. You know who I am, but I do not think that we know one another well. I am sorry that I have not had the chance to get to know you better, but maybe in the future that will happen.

'I believe that you wrote me some letters. I know that you claim that you did not do this, but I think that there is enough evidence to satisfy me, at least, that it was you.

'I am writing now to say sorry to you. The only reason why anybody should have written those letters was that I – and my assistant, Mma Makutsi – must have done something in the past to make you feel angry with us. If we have done that – and I do not know what it could be – then I want you to know that I am very sorry for making you feel that way about us. You should not have written to us in the way you did, but I am still saying sorry for anything we have done, Mma, and I am asking you to accept that apology.

'I think, by the way, that I knew your aunt, the one who lived for some years in Mochudi and is now late. Sephotho is not a common name, so my late friend must have been your relative. I remember that she always spoke very highly of one of her nieces who was doing very well in Gaborone, and that must have been you! Your aunt was very proud of you, as I recall.

'Yours sincerely, Precious Ramotswe.'

Mma Ramotswe finished. She lifted her gaze up, to find Mma Makutsi, her pencil suspended in mid-air, staring at her. 'You can't say that, Mma Ramotswe. Violet Sephotho is—'

'Is a woman like you and me, Mma,' said Mma Ramotswe. 'Who can feel bad about herself, the same as everyone. And who wants to be loved, the same as everyone. So saying what I have just said is better, far better, than making her feel even less loved than she is.'

She looked at Mma Makutsi, whose pencil still remained poised. 'Did you get all of that, Mma Makutsi?'

The pencil descended again to the notepad and made further squiggles across the page.

'We won't hear again from Violet Sephotho,' said Mma Ramotswe quietly. 'That is the end of that.'

She paused. She could see that Mma Makutsi was not convinced.

'You don't agree?' Mma Ramotswe asked.

Mma Makutsi shook her head. 'Why will she stop? There is something that made her do that. That something will not have gone away.'

'Yes, there is something that made her do it,' Mma Ramotswe said. 'It is called envy, and it can make people do very strange things, Mma. She is envious of you because you have everything that she does not. You did so well at the Botswana Secretarial College with your ninety-seven per cent. How does a fifty per cent—'

'At the most,' interjected Mma Makutsi. 'Sometimes even less. Forty-two per cent once, I think.'

'There you are,' said Mma Ramotswe. She knew how hard it had been for Mma Makutsi: the younger woman had started with so little, had fought for everything she had; had lived with her bad skin, with her large glasses, lived with everything. And even now that she had something which many women would dearly love – a kind husband, or almost, with his own business – she could not believe that anybody would be envious of her.

'It's your Phuti too,' said Mma Ramotswe. 'He has given you a position, security. Violet has none of that and she resents you for it. She wants to put you down. That's why she wrote.'

'But she wrote to you, Mma Ramotswe. Your name was on the envelope.'

'Of course she did. That is because that would cover her tracks. She wrote to me and had you in her sights at the same time. I would probably be just as bad in her eyes. Good husband. A nice house. Cattle.' She paused. 'And that is why we must answer her hatred with love. I can't say whether it will change her in her heart – it probably won't. But if it makes her feel even just a little bit better about herself, she will be less envious.'

Mma Makutsi laid aside her pencil and stared across the room at her employer. She opened her mouth to speak, but then closed it again. There was much she wanted to say, but even these few moments of contemplation of what Mma Ramotswe had said had shown her that everything that she, Mma Makutsi, would have said was wrong. Mma Ramotswe was right: evil repaid with retribution, with punishment, had achieved half its goal; evil repaid with kindness was shown to be what it really was, a small, petty thing, not something frightening at all, but something pitiable, a paltry affair. So she picked up her pencil, opened a drawer in her desk, and dropped the pencil inside. 'I think you're probably right, Mma,' she said, through tight lips. 'You usually are in these matters, because you are a kind lady. But I wish that you were wrong. Which you aren't. But I still wish it.'

The letter to Violet was an easy task by comparison with what now lay before Mma Ramotswe. She had managed to contact Mma Sebina by telephone and had told her that she needed to see her with some important information.

'About my brother?' asked Mma Sebina brightly. 'He is coming to see me tonight. We are going to go to the cinema together.'

Mma Ramotswe swallowed. If she were to be completely honest, then the answer to that would be no, it is not about your brother, because he is not your brother. But she could not; the truth could be too cruel on occasion, and this was one such. And yet that same truth would have to be disclosed very soon.

'It is about your brother,' she said. 'Yes, it is, Mma.'

And now she was standing in front of Mma Sebina's gate and calling out *Ko! Ko!* And there was Mma Sebina coming out of her front door, wiping her hands on a piece of kitchen towel, and waving to her.

'Mma Ramotswe! You must come in and try what I have just baked. Some banana bread, Mma. It's a special recipe. Kenneth told me he liked it.'

'Kenneth?'

'My brother. That is his first name. Kenneth Sekape.'

Mma Ramotswe looked down at the ground, and Mma Sebina noticed.

'Is there something wrong?' There was panic in her voice. 'There's something wrong, Mma. Oh, you have come to give me bad news . . .'

She started to wail, the wail of the bereaved, the widow, that heart-rending inimitable cry that signified the sudden, overwhelming onset of a grief. Mma Ramotswe reached forward and seized Mma Sebina by the arm, pulling her towards her. 'No, Mma! It is not that! Mr Sekape is all right. It is not that, Mma.'

Mma Sebina strangled her cries. She stared mutely at Mma Ramotswe. 'Then . . .'

Mma Ramotswe shook her head, as if trying to make sense of some confusion within her. 'It is all my fault. I should have checked up on what Mma Potokwani told me. She has too much to remember, Mma. She can get things mixed up.'

Mma Sebina frowned. 'What is mixed up?'

Mma Ramotswe took a deep breath. Now, very suddenly, she felt herself acutely aware of where she was – standing in front of Mma Sebina's house, under a sky from which the rain clouds had cleared and which was now empty, blue, limitless. And across which a bird of prey was describing huge, lazy circles. She thought it strange that at a moment like this one should notice such things, but she had heard that one did; as a person facing death may suddenly find that he is looking at some humdrum object in his room, and seeing its beauty.

'Mr Sekape is not really your brother, I'm afraid, Mma. Mma Potokwani got things mixed up.' She would tell her in due course that there had been a brother and that he was late. Now was not the time, though, as she had caused Mma Sebina quite enough distress already.

Mma Ramotswe had half expected another wail, and was prepared for it. Instead she saw an expression of curiosity come over the other woman's face. It was curiosity, but it was also a look of pleasurable discovery, as if the information that had just been given to her was not disappointing but welcome.

'So he is not my brother,' she said.

'No. He is not. I'm so sorry, Mma.'

Mma Sebina fingered the crumpled piece of kitchen towel that she had been carrying. 'I am glad about that,' she said.

It took a moment or two, but then the realisation came to Mma Ramotswe. Of course, of course. 'Oh, Mma,' she said. 'I'm sorry that he proved to be one of those men who have a low opinion of women. I knew it was going to be difficult for you. I knew it. So, yes, you must be glad that such a man is not your brother.'

Mma Sebina looked at her in puzzlement. 'But he does like women,' she said. 'He said that he liked me very much. And . . .'

'Yes?'

'Well, Mma Ramotswe. What you have told me is very good news because . . . well, because I like Kenneth very much. I like him . . . more than one would normally like a brother. Well, more as one would like a man who might become a husband. Of course I could not think that while he was still my brother, and I thought that he would just be a very good friend. But now . . .'

'And what about him?'

Mma Sebina looked away. 'I think that he will be pleased too, Mma. I think he will be very pleased.'

Mma Ramotswe felt the tension of the meeting ebb away. She had expected it to be painful and instead it had become an occasion of pleasure, of complicity in a future romance.

Mma Sebina now took Mma Ramotswe by the arm and steered her towards the door. 'Let us go and try some of that banana bread, Mma,' she said. And then she added: 'It's strange, isn't it? I consulted you to find me a family, and you went out and found me a husband.'

Mma Ramotswe smiled at this. It seemed a bit premature for Mma Sebina to be thinking in terms of marrying Mr Sekape, but one thing was very clear: she was a woman with a mission, and in Mma Ramotswe's view, women with a mission usually achieved it, as many men in Botswana – and elsewhere, she imagined – had found out.

Over the cup of tea and the generous slice of banana bread, Mma Ramotswe tackled the last matter that she knew she had to raise with Mma Sebina. It was simpler, now that the information about the mistake had been so easily dealt with, but it would still require tact.

'There is something else I know, Mma,' she said. 'There is something about the reason why you were taken in by Mma Potokwani in the first place. I have found that out and I think that you may want to know it.'

'About my mother?' said Mma Sebina.

'Yes. It is about your mother.'

Mma Sebina lowered her eyes. 'Is it something that—' She broke off. Then: 'Would it make me feel bad about her?'

Mma Ramotswe thought about this. 'It might,' she said. 'But if you knew this thing, it would still be possible for you to forgive her.'

'Even though she is late? She is late, isn't she?'

Mma Ramotswe nodded. 'She is late. But it is still possible to forgive people who are late, you know. It's important to do that sometimes.'

'Then I forgive her,' said Mma Sebina. 'I forgive my mother for . . .'

'For . . .'

Mma Sebina raised a hand. 'No, please don't tell me, Mma. I would prefer not to know. And I forgive her whatever it is, even if I do not know.'

'Then I am sure that wherever she is, she is pleased, Mma. I am sure, by the way, that she loved you a great deal. And I am sure that the thing that happened was not something she would have wished to happen.'

'I am sure that is true,' said Mma Sebina.

They drank their tea. There is a final thing, Mma Ramotswe suddenly thought; a final, final thing. The woman who had kept a chair in the tree: why had she been so adamant that Mma Sebina was not adopted? She claimed, after all, to have witnessed her birth; why would she have said that?

'There was a friend of your mother,' said Mma Ramotswe. 'I saw her when I went down to Otse. She has a tree—'

'And a chair hanging up in the tree?' interrupted Mma Sebina. 'Oh dear.'

'Why do you say that, Mma?'

'Because that poor lady lives in a world of dreams,' said Mma Sebina. 'She is famous for that. And if she told you that she used to have a tomato stall, and that the Minister of Agriculture awarded her a prize for the tomatoes – that is all nonsense, Mma. I'm sorry to say. All nonsense. But she's harmless and if she wants to sit under that tree with the chair hanging in it, then there are worse ways of spending one's time.'

Mma Ramotswe had to agree with this. There were. Considerably worse ways.

Mr J. L. B. Matekoni arrived home the following morning, unannounced. Mma Ramotswe had not expected him until the next afternoon, but his truck pulled up outside the gate while Mma Ramotswe was taking her early morning walk about the garden. The plants were doing well with the recent rains, and she was examining a shrub which she had planted a few days before, and thinking about Mma Makutsi, when she heard the horn sound and she looked up to see his truck.

She ran towards the gate. He waved from the cab, and so did Motholeli, sitting beside him. Then she pulled the gate open and the truck passed through. She saw the layer of dust on the window through which Motholeli looked at her, smiling. She saw the spattering of red mud thrown up against the mudguards; they had travelled through rain.

Mr J. L. B. Matekoni stepped out. 'We left very early,' he said. 'I woke up at three and I decided that we would leave then. It is easier driving in the cool of the day.'

'Of course.' She looked at his face, searching. She knew the answer, but she still looked. People had sometimes defied the worst predictions of medical science; it had happened.

He dropped his gaze to the ground, and she knew. She knew immediately.

'I'm sorry, Rra.'

His lips moved slightly, but she could not hear what he was saying. She glanced at Motholeli through the mud-streaked glass; she was stuffing something into a bag; she was absorbed.

'And how is she dealing with this?' Mma Ramotswe whispered.

Mr J. L. B. Matekoni looked up at her, and she saw that his eyes were moist. Men can cry. Mechanics. Any man.

'She is being very brave. It's as if nothing has happened.' His voice broke off for a moment. Then, 'She says that it was worth going. That she is glad that we tried.'

Mma Ramotswe nodded. 'I will help her out of the truck,' she said. 'You must be very tired. You go in and have a shower. All that dust, Rra. All that dust.'

There was much to do. Motholeli was insistent that she wanted to get back to school that morning, in spite of having got up so early. 'I want to see my friends again,' she said. 'I want to tell them about Johannesburg.'

After breakfast, Mma Ramotswe helped her into the tiny white van and loaded the wheelchair in the back. Then she drove off to the school and parked outside the main gate. They were early and there were no children about, just the man who swept the playground, moving slowly backwards and forwards, his brush raising a small cloud of dust with each stroke. Along the line of the gate, the grass, encouraged into growth by the heavy rains, was dark green, lush.

They sat there, waiting for other children to arrive.

'That grass,' said Mma Ramotswe, pointing to the fence. 'Look at it. That would keep some cattle very happy. But there are no cattle in town these days. I remember when there were, you know. Lots of cattle. People just brought them into town with them to keep an eye on them. And I remember when we had telephones that everybody had to share – if you were lucky enough to have a telephone in the first place – party lines. When you spoke, other people could pick up their phone and listen too. You had to be careful.'

'I would not have liked that,' said Motholeli.

'You got used to it,' said Mma Ramotswe. 'You can get used to anything, you know.' She had not intended to say that, and it was only afterwards that she realised that Motholeli might have misunderstood her, might have taken it badly. You can get used to anything – even a wheelchair, not being able to walk, even that. She had not meant to say it.

She glanced sideways at the little girl. Motholeli was looking at her hands, examining her fingernails.

'I am used to it now, Mma. I am used to . . . what has happened to me. You must not worry about me.'

Mma Ramotswe reached out and put a hand on her knee. 'I did not want you to go. I was worried that it would come to nothing. I wasn't at all sure about that doctor.'

'He tried,' said Motholeli. 'And the people in Johannesburg tried too. They had all sorts of machines. But then they said that they could not do anything. I heard them. They said it to Mr J. L. B. Matekoni, but I overheard them. And he was crying.'

'Mr J. L. B. Matekoni was crying?'

'Yes. He was.' She finished her examination of her nails and began to wind down the car window. 'I don't want anybody to cry for me. There is no need. I am happy. I will carry on being happy.'

A small boy on a bicycle had now arrived at the front gate. He dismounted with grave caution; the bicycle, gleaming in the morning sunlight, was brand new.

'Look at him,' said Motholeli. 'He is very proud of his bicycle.'

'Yes,' said Mma Ramotswe. 'He is proud.' She turned to Motholeli. 'And I am proud too, Motholeli. I am a very, very proud lady.'

When she returned to Zebra Drive, she found Mr J. L. B. Matekoni still sitting at the kitchen table, the breakfast plates all about him. He had the air of a man who had been defeated over something, who had been proved wrong.

'So,' she said. 'That is over.'

He did not look at her, but traced a pattern on the table-cloth with a finger. 'I'm sorry, Mma,' he said. 'You were right. I should not have believed those people. And I still have to pay them. I have taken a loan. It is very bad.'

She looked at him, this man whose generous heart she had never doubted once, not once, in all the time she had known him; this man who had become her husband and of whom she was so proud.

'No, there is no need for a loan,' she said gently. 'I have sold cattle. There is easily enough money.'

'I cannot . . .'

'You can. She is my child too.'

He raised his head; there was so much in his eyes, she thought: disappointment, embarrassment, regret – and tired-ness too. 'I was stupid to believe that a miracle might be possible. I was so foolish.'

Mma Ramotswe sat down at the table and took his hand. 'It is not at all foolish to hope for miracles,' she said. 'No, it is not foolish, Rra. Not foolish at all. There are many miracles.'

He asked her what she meant, and she explained. There had been a miracle at Speedy Motors while he was away. A woman had looked for somebody to be her family and she had found him. That was a miracle. And Mma Makutsi had paid tribute to Charlie – was that not another miracle? And there had been these life-giving rains, which had made Botswana turn from brown to green and would make the cattle fat within days. All of these were miracles, were they not? Of course one might still wish for further miracles. There was that ominous knocking sound in the tiny white van; if that were to vanish, then that would be another most welcome miracle.

But one had to be careful, Mma Ramotswe reminded herself: one should not ask for too many things in this life, especially when one already had so much.